The Reluctant Patient: A Journey of Trust

The Reluctant Patient:
A Journey of Trust

Ian G. Wallis

Winchester, UK
Washington, USA

First published by Circle Books, 2014

Circle Books is an imprint of John Hunt Publishing Ltd., Laurel House, Station Approach, Alresford, Hants, SO24 9JH, UK
office1@jhpbooks.net
www.johnhuntpublishing.com
www.circle-books.com

For distributor details and how to order please visit the 'Ordering' section on our website.

Text copyright: Ian G. Wallis 2013

ISBN: 978 1 78279 673 2

A CIP catalogue record for this book is available from the British Library.

Design: Stuart Davies

Printed in the USA by Edwards Brothers Malloy

We operate a distinctive and ethical publishing philosophy in all areas of our business, from our global network of authors to production and worldwide distribution.

CONTENTS

To members of the
Northern Ordination Course, 2007–8,
as well as
to the church communities
of St Michael & All Angels, Houghton-le-Spring,
and St Mark, Broomhill, Sheffield.

For keeping faith
and carrying on,
thank you.

Preface

One of the injustices of life is that time cheats on us. Although it's supposed to pass at a constant rate, experience tells us otherwise. It flies by when we're enjoying ourselves, ticks over through life's routines and almost grinds to a halt when encountering circumstances we would rather escape from at the earliest opportunity. For most of us, illness belongs firmly within the final time zone as life is put on hold whilst we suffer some malfunction or alien invasion.

But does illness have to be experienced in this way – a source of inconvenience and diminishment? Or can it, at least in certain circumstances, create space for us to embrace fresh appreciations capable of enriching our lives as a whole? This brief volume chronicles one journey, undertaken by a reluctant patient, from the former outlook towards the latter.

Self-evidently, this book wouldn't have been written if I had remained fine and dandy, yet it seems incongruous to thank a failing body for precipitating a text. Yet there were many who helped me to recognise that, for all its uncertainties and depletions, illness can yield blessing. We need not name them here for their contributions animate this volume. In truth, what follows is an extended appreciation.

More people than I can remember have heard or read sections of this manuscript and encouraged me to make it more generally available. In particular, Stephen Cherry and Martin Kerry generously agreed to comment on the full manuscript, offering valuable feedback. To everyone who has participated in this labour, thank you.

I am indebted to Jim Cotter for granting permission to include an excerpt from *Healing – More or Less* (Cairns Publications, 1990). Similarly, to the trustees of Julia Darling's Estate to cite from one of Julia's poems, 'Chemotherapy', published in *Sudden*

Collapses in Public Places (Arc, 2003), as well as to Bloodaxe Books Ltd to incorporate a poem by ASJ Tessimond, 'Saving Grace', published in his *Collected Poems* (Bloodaxe, 2010). Biblical quotations are from the *New Revised Standard Version*, Anglicized Edition, copyright © 1989, 1995.

And, finally, to Liz and Tess, companions through life, source of joy and consolation.

Chapter I

Out of the Blue

"Are we going to watch *Atonement* or not?" It was New Year's Eve in Edinburgh, UK, and Hogmanay celebrations were still some hours away. Liz and I pondered whether to take in the screen version of Ian McEwan's novel. "Not before you've phoned the *National Health Service Advice Line (NHS 24),*" came her resolute reply. Reluctantly, I conceded.

Several weeks before Christmas, I had gone down with a severe cold which developed into a chest infection. There was nothing dramatic. No sudden deterioration or worsening in condition, just a gradual decline that could readily be accommodated within the ebb and flow of minor ailments accompanying most of us through life. The dog walking, though, set me thinking. Every morning around six, Tess (our golden retriever) and I embark on an hour's exercise. Our normal pace is more than a walk but less than a canter, a spirited trot enabling us to cover a couple of miles or so before returning for tea and toast, although Tess majors on the latter.

Recently, though, the tempo dropped significantly to little more than a totter and a pretty unstable one at that. It felt as if I had been switched into slow motion or slipped some speed-inhibiting drug. Each step was shallow and laboured as the whole operation became more like a punishment to endure than an outing to enjoy. "Why should this be?" I wondered. Even so, the 'chest infection' theory seemed as good an explanation as any. And there was always the toast, that universal remedy which, when administered with lashings of butter and marmalade, spreads a layer of comfort over most of life's ills.

The *NHS 24* telephonist who answered was courteous and helpful. No automated message, no choice of options, a real person. Although not medically qualified, she was reassuring with her careful attention, sympathetic responses and promise of a return call within the hour. There was none of the pre-recorded "Your call is important to us" condescension. Instead, someone who seemed sufficiently interested to invest in our encounter. And it is surprising what can be communicated between those who, however briefly, choose to be present in the present for one another.

Well before the sixty minutes had elapsed my mobile rang and, once again, I was greeted by the animated tones of a Scottish accent, this time those of a nurse consultant. We quickly established a rapport as she proceeded to gather symptoms with commensurate ease: shortage of breath, chronic fatigue, cold sweats, tightness in the chest, poor concentration. Then there were the minor heart abnormalities that had first emerged thirty years previously when, wired up to an exercise bicycle monitoring pulse rate, it began to emit a string of high-pitched bleeps more reminiscent of Morse code than a heart rhythm.

As far as I was concerned, none of these symptoms alone gave rise to concern. They were isolated skirmishes containable by the body's defences without intervention, especially if calling for reinforcements entailed eking out space in an overfull diary to visit a GP. But once assembled they seemed more menacing and potent, capable of mounting an assault and inflicting damage. Seen together they demanded attention.

This is precisely what they received. The phone line fell silent as my advisor, once appraised of the situation, consulted a colleague before returning to the air. "Mr Wallis?" "That's me." "There's an ambulance on its way to take you to the nearest hospital for further investigations." Now the silence was of my making as I attempted to process the import of her instructions. Ambulance, further investigations – what about the multiplex cinema and seeing in the New Year? My surprise must have been palpable because, before managing a response, she proffered an explanation.

What struck me was how readily she concluded that something was amiss once the symptoms were brought together. But there is the rub. I didn't, and my guess is I am not unusual in this respect. We can become so preoccupied with the pressures of the moment that there is little space to process those minor disturbances that frequently impede progress and invade our days. We can lack the motivation also, for the process of reflection is not simply a drain on resources, it has the potential to disturb our equilibrium by uncovering things we would rather ignore.

For me, health issues readily fall into this category. Through the years, no doubt resulting from early exposure to a strict and life-negating form of Christianity, I have tended to view my body as a lazy mule requiring correction or a flighty stallion in need of taming. Either way, it is an adversarial relationship in which one part of me pits itself against another. I suspect many of us with demanding jobs and lifestyles have become adept at disciplining the flesh to squeeze a little more into each day, or at developing strategies for drowning out its protests when pushed too far. In the thick of things, we appear to have little choice given the levels of expectation and workload surrounding us; but, as I was about to discover, every so often our bodies stage a coup d'état.

Hailing an ambulance, though, still seemed excessive. Why couldn't Liz drive me to the nearest hospital? After all, it wasn't as if I needed urgent medical attention. Suddenly, a chasm opened up between my home-made diagnosis and the one entertained by my medical advisor. It left me disturbed and uncertain. Had I misread the symptoms? Was this 'belt and braces' approach a NHS ruse to reduce insurance liability? Or was I *really* ill? For all that, I still didn't warm to the prospect of flashing lights and sirens.

Although there is a pronounced public dimension to my vocation as a Christian minister, I have never found being 'on show' easy. It is not in my nature to seek the limelight which, no doubt, explains why the prospect of blazing along the streets of Scotland's capital in an ambulance didn't appeal. Cars pulling over, running red lights, people stopping to stare – what a lot of fuss about nothing. There was comfort in the knowledge that my identity would remain hidden behind darkened glass. Mine would be an anonymous presence. Come to think of it, not so unlike the other time most of us are transported publicly against our wishes; although on that occasion, hopefully we are beyond caring!

Once my therapeutic phone-line encounter with *NHS 24* was over, the countdown to the paramedics' arrival commenced. But what to do? In an instant, my head filled with questions. What about this evening's celebrations? Would I need an overnight bag? How should I break the news? When did I last change my undies? Is my will up to date? My mind oscillated between trivia and the essential before Liz, returning to the room, rescued me from my preoccupations. "What did they say?" It was a straightforward question, but one that flummoxed me. Searching for an answer, I heard myself saying, "*Atonement* will have to wait, we're off to *Accident and Emergency* instead."

It suddenly struck me how difficult it is to share unwelcome news, especially with those closest to us. For one thing, it requires us to admit to being at the mercy of factors beyond our control. Such exposure can be so emotionally demanding that we are tempted to retreat into a kind of imaginary world where we are masters of our destiny. At some point, though, reality has a habit of impressing itself upon us, forcing us to confront an uncomfortable truth, namely that our lives are inextricably linked to persons and circumstances beyond our manipulation or making.

For another, we would rather spare our nearest and dearest from having to join us in the turbulent waters threatening to overwhelm. Instinctively, I wanted to reassure Liz that all was well. That everything was going according to plan. That our feet were firmly planted upon *terra firma* or, at the very least, that we were safe within a lifeboat able to ride the storm. But my face revealed a different reality, expressing a level of honesty I lacked the courage to articulate. Faces possess that capacity, to turn us inside out. Whilst most of us become adept at using ours to mask the person within, vulnerability, like many forms of suffering, strips away the superficial to reveal the naked self.

Paradoxically, it was here, in this 'communion of the vulnerable', that genuine encounter became possible. As our eyes met, a reassuring sense of stability returned as the covenant between us embraced the chaos of the moment. Superficially, nothing had changed, but at a profound level I found myself in a different place – confronting an unknown future within the security of an enduring love.

No sooner had that moment of transfiguration passed than panic flooded back in. What shall I wear? Should I brush my teeth? Who supplies the Lucozade? It felt as if I urgently needed to prepare for something without being sure what it was, like those stressful dreams in which we can never quite make it to where we are supposed to be or, if we do, we feel humiliated because of being inappropriately attired. My mind darted back to those wintry early morning walks when I would don layers of thermal clothing and Tess wore nothing save her birthday suit. Then I recalled those haunting words rehearsed at funerals, "We brought nothing into the world and it is certain we can carry nothing out," which pressed home the seriousness of my predicament.

It was an unsettling sensation, tinged with apprehension and adventure as I prepared to embark on what felt like a blind date with the Grim Reaper equipped with little more than a credit card and a tube of toothpaste. It all seemed surreal, but there was nothing other-worldly about the door buzzer. Glimpsing through the curtains it became apparent my carriage had arrived.

Chapter 2

How Inconvenient!

"I need this like a hole in the head!" Inconvenience was my overarching mindset on leaving the apartment. Inconvenience tinged with irritation. I had so been looking forward to meeting up with old friends to bring in the New Year. Then there were those work-related tasks clamouring for attention tomorrow and beyond. All of this was suddenly put on hold by some gate-crasher who had muscled its way into my diary. Someone needed to take responsibility and apologise. But who? Whose fault was it? Who was to blame?

I had often reflected on this when working as a parish priest; how many of us find ourselves entertaining such sentiments at times of illness or distress, along with that sense of being held to account or punished for some former misdemeanour. "What have I done to deserve this?" seems strangely anachronistic within a world of science and technology claiming to have banished interventions of celestial overseers charged with administering justice to the errant and unruly.

Yet such protests persist. They reflect, I think, a desire to impose a measure of order on to what would otherwise be a dangerously unpredictable world. The rationale, although rarely articulated, goes something like this. Surely, bad things cannot happen to good people? So, if they do, there must be a good reason for it. And, in the absence of a more plausible explanation, the ancient law of *lex talionis* immortalised in the Gilbert and Sullivan lyric, "Let the punishment fit the crime," continues to hold sway. You might think this offers little comfort, but I suppose it is infinitely preferable to inhabiting a capricious, amoral universe where keeping on the 'straight and narrow' offers no insurance against life's misfortunes.

We also long to survive. When our lives are endangered in some way, instinctively we explore all possible escape routes. Again, there is a subliminal dimension at play which circumvents conscious thought. One expression of this childlike (not childish) response is to cry out, believing there is a parent-like God 'out there' who is able to save us. We petition, plead, even negotiate, without any real sense of the enormity of what we are asking or even of whether there is 'anyone' listening who is able to come to our aid. The biblical book of Psalms is replete with expressions of this most natural of predispositions:

> Incline your ear to me; rescue me speedily... Turn, O Lord, save my life; deliver me for the sake of your steadfast love... Save me from the mouth of the lion! From the horns of the wild oxen you have rescued me. I will tell of your name to my brothers and sisters; in the midst of the congregation I will praise you... I cry to you; save me, that I may observe your decrees...
> – Psalm 31.2; 6.4; 22.21–22; 119.146

Moving downstairs, I was aware of an inner voice expressing these concerns – "Why me?" "Give me another chance!" "Help!" "Get me out of here!" – but it lacked intensity. For some reason, I wasn't preoccupied with eleventh hour confessions or plea bargaining, less still with making a heaven-bound 999 rescue call. There seemed little point. In its place, an overwhelming conviction that any influence I might once have exerted over my life had been relinquished and now rested elsewhere. I was at the mercy of forces beyond my creating and circumstances outside of my control – weak and powerless.

It was a conviction that intensified the moment I crossed the threshold into the back of the ambulance. In an instant, my new identity emerged. No longer was I a member of the general public. I had become a patient! It is an interesting word and one defining the estate it conveys. Patient, like patience, derives from the Latin for suffering. To be a patient is to be a sufferer – one who is done to and who, under the influence of something or someone, exhibits sufferance.

Illness is an obvious case in point. I had not knowingly courted my symptoms nor was I able to eradicate them. They exerted a hold on me and a debilitating one at that, leaving me little option but to grin and bear it. Yet, paradoxically, calling upon paramedics and their colleagues entailed further suffering of a kind, not only in the sense of enduring whatever pain or discomfort would be associated with administering treatment, but also and more fundamentally because I was about to entrust my life into their hands. It is no coincidence that medics are accused of 'playing god'; in truth, sometimes we need them to.

One thing I have come to appreciate through ministering as a priest is the difference between being a *patient* and a *victim*. Clearly, there is common ground; and without oversimplifying matters, to be a patient is to endure suffering without being obliterated by it, whereas victims are consumed by their condition. There is, I think, an important distinction here and one revolving around how we relate to suffering in its many manifestations. Whether it takes us over to the extent that our identity as persons becomes subsumed within it or whether we are able to maintain a measure of independence – inner space to be ourselves and to determine, to some measure, suffering's impact upon us.

For me, this is where faith comes in – a capacity to relate beyond our immediate circumstances, drawing us out of ourselves in search of a fuller sense of personhood. Faith that is a kind of vulnerability not only to the suffering threatening to overwhelm us, but also to a profounder reality transcending the present moment with all its pain, fear and uncertainty. A tenacious faith capable of rescuing us from becoming victims against our wills.

Once settled on the stretcher, I was content to place my trust in the paramedics. "Please remove your top," seemed an innocuous request and one I readily acceded to despite the near zero temperature outside. I was slightly baffled, though, by the emergence of a razor from a storage tray. How would the removal of my beard further clinical investigations? I pondered. All became clear when clumps of hair started disappearing from my chest to ensure firm contact for the sticky sensors of the ECG monitor. I first came across this piece of apparatus recording the electrical activity of the heart in my early twenties after the 'exercise bike' incident when an ectopic heartbeat had been identified (more of that later). In those days, rubber suckers applied with generous helpings of KY Gel were employed which made a habit of popping off just as the technician attempted to obtain a reading. You can imagine the ensuing pandemonium!

There was no plunger work on this occasion, just shaving, sticking and wiring for sound. As with the *NHS 24* staff, I was impressed by the manner of the paramedics, conveying a sense of reassurance and trustworthiness. It caused me to reflect on the importance of human interaction within the healing process, those 'soft' components so easily overlooked within an increasingly technology-rich, target-driven approach to health care. After all, how do you measure the therapeutic benefit of a kind word, a considerate gesture, an affirming smile? Yet few of us would deny that personal encounter, whatever the context, is immeasurably impoverished without such graces. This is no hankering after the 'good old days' when nurses devoted their time to bedside niceties such as mopping fevered brows and holding timorous hands. It is, rather, an acknowledgement that trust is established within the healing dynamic as much by the quality of relating as by the demonstration of technical competence.

The time of reckoning had arrived. Suitably connected, the LCD display recording pulse and blood pressure, together with my heart trace, began to reveal their secrets. I noticed the easy, relaxed manner of my attendants changed, becoming strained and awkward. This caused me to check the monitor – 130, 40, 50, 60, 70, 180. This time my pulse looked more like a darts score! I knew from past experience that a resting pulse in the high hundreds signalled trouble as did the findings of the ECG, revealing my normal heart rhythm had been replaced by a rapid, intermittent and shallow pattern. Any sign of regular operation had disappeared.

Little diagnosis was necessary. The evidence spoke for itself as the training of my medical companions kicked in. First, a high dose aspirin placed under my tongue, then a cannula was expertly inserted into the back of my hand in preparation for administering drugs intravenously. The ECG trace was relayed via mobile phone to the nearest hospital yielding the predictable response, "Bring him in."

My mind flitted back to Corporal Jones of *Dad's Army* fame who, during times of impending danger, would exclaim, "Don't panic, don't panic," whilst doing precisely the opposite. There was little to be gained by maintaining all was well and that we were simply embarking on a sightseeing tour of Edinburgh's notable infirmaries. There was too much honesty around and, in a perverse sort of way, I appreciated it. 'Ignorance is bliss' has little to commend it at times such as these and I have often wondered whether the strategy of keeping patients in the dark about their prognosis to spare them unnecessary hardship is, although well-meaning, misguided. In one sense, it does reduce anxiety and fearfulness; but, in another, such deception (for that is what it amounts to) can deepen the experience of power-lessness and isolation as patients are left to suffer alone within a climate of half-truths and pretence where that love capable of "bearing all things... enduring all things" struggles to be present (cf 1 Corinthians, chapter 13).

If ignorance and pretence had little to commend them, injecting a high dose of stress-inducing angst into the system didn't seem an appealing alternative. Instead, the airwaves filled with voices making arrangements or collecting medical history interspersed with periods of intense silence. I was keenly aware that my condition was dangerous, potentially life threatening unless treated as a matter of urgency. Yet, for all that, I wasn't preoccupied with regret at life being cut short or with guilt over unfinished business or relationships compromised by something I had said or done. All this seemed secondary to ensuring there was opportunity to say farewell to Liz.

But what would I say? What words could bear the weight of parting? Back in 1990, I had the privilege of nursing my mother at home during what proved to be her final months as lung cancer progressed relentlessly towards its predicable conclusion. As the end approached, she spent most of the time unconscious or in a curious hinterland between this life and what appeared to be the next. One moment she would be conversing with deceased relatives only, awaking abruptly, to find herself in the company of Father and me. On this occasion, Mother hadn't stirred for a number of days. Suddenly she regained consciousness and announced, "I'm dying now." Father and I looked at one another, our minds as desolate as our complexions. We struggled to say anything. Words seemed so inadequate, so redundant, so incapable of accompanying the enormity of the moment.

Things were little different in the ambulance. Not knowing how long the window of opportunity would be, I forced myself to string something together: "Thank you, forgive me, keep faith, abide in our love."

Speeding along to the screech of sirens, strapped to a stretcher, connected to various devices as a concoction of drugs was being injected into my bloodstream, I became alarmingly aware of just how tenuous my hold on life was. I felt totally dependent upon health professionals, medicines and diagnostic apparatus of which I had no personal knowledge. Time did not permit inquiring into their probity or clinical effectiveness. Even if it had, I doubt whether it would have made a jot of difference. What was called for on my part could not be reached through in-depth analysis or personal scrutiny – a radical trust transcending intellectual judgement and emotional response. A form of 'letting go', risky, placing me at the mercy of realities beyond my beckoning, where evidence of whether such a personal investment was well-placed would only emerge beyond the point of no return.

Chapter 3

An Emergency Case?

After participating in what felt like a cross-country rally, we screeched to a halt outside the main entrance to the *Accident and Emergency* department. The rear doors opened. Immediately, we embarked on the next leg speeding through a bustling waiting room, brimming with injuries and complaints, whilst dodging patients preoccupied by plasma TVs. Weaving our way through the crowd, there was a furious exchange of medical jargon across the stretcher which, although largely incomprehensible, I assumed was about me.

Rather than requesting a translation, I took a moment to overcome my guilt and savour that 'jumping the queue' feeling – one of the few perks of being a stretcher case, I thought, particularly appreciated by us English who are programmed 'to take our turn'. But the sensation was short lived, for once ensconced within the holding ward, I took my place amongst the backlog of emergency cases!

At this juncture, the paramedics gestured their readiness to leave. Not for the first time that evening I found myself struggling for words. After all, what do you say to someone in such circumstances – to those anonymous persons about whom we know little and yet who leave a lasting impression upon us owing to the nature and intensity of the encounter? Scanning the recesses of a faltering mind, I rapidly exhausted options before resorting to the only container remotely capable of conveying the weight of my appreciation, "Thank you."

"That's OK, we're just doing our jobs." It was a well-rehearsed and predictable reply. Yet, as we exchanged glances, I sensed these words meant something. That what motivated these lifesavers extended beyond earning a living and touched a deeper vein, a sense of vocation, of being caught up in a profounder drama where they had been given a role to fulfil and one whose value resided not so much in a monthly pay cheque as in the satisfaction it engendered in those who made it their own. Nothing more was said. Nothing needed to be.

In the moments that followed I mused on the limits of language. How, for all the ways in which it enriches life, under-pinning our capacity for thought, expression and communi-cation, it is readily muted by those extremes of human experience which stretch beyond its semantic reach. Those concentrated intensities of living when we instinctively draw on other capac-ities – the inarticulate registers of our voices, the involuntary movements of our bodies, embracing with our arms, eyes or lips and, of course, those eloquent silences occupying the moment without interpretation or response. Encountering grace is surely one of those occasions when we are rendered speechless by some act of generosity or kindness. All we can do is receive it for the gift that it is. And, as I was coming to realise, such receptivity characterises the patient's lot.

The sound of apparatus wending its way towards my bedside returned me to the present. On arrival, various accessories were put in place – a cuff to the upper arm, a strange looking thermometer under my tongue and what appeared to be a clothes peg on the crown of my index finger. Each measured some key bodily function (although it wasn't always obvious how!) before results were dutifully logged in what I came to think of as my *Book of Life*, a blue loose-leaf folder housed at the foot of the bed containing my vital statistics which would be checked and updated on a regular basis. Then more stickers – ankles, wrists and around the heart like points on a compass – which looked remarkably similar to the set applied in the ambulance before being discarded along with vestiges of a once hairy chest. Judging from the sharp intake of breath and furtive glance to confirm I was still in the land of the living, this latest ECG reading confirmed the paramedics' suspicions. It was then I realised no one was about to sound the false alarm and reassure me that the precautionary strategy of *NHS 24* had been a well-meaning overreaction. All was not well – 12/31 was about to become my 9/11.

The ensuing veil of despond was temporarily lifted by the arrival of the next chariot, the tea trolley, steered by a jolly Glaswegian dressed in another colour and style of uniform who plied us with weak, lukewarm beverages accompanied by those ubiquitous *rich tea* biscuits which were dispensed with the same degree of precision as a prescription drug. Hardly the Hogmanay fare I had envisaged earlier in the day, but nonetheless welcome, not least because it was administered without a needle.

My experience as a priest had taught me that 'tea and sympathy' was a reassuring remedy in times of distress. But I had often wondered why? Was it the preoccupying business of brewing or the undemanding nature of an infusion which can be readily fortified with sugar or something stronger? Perhaps the active ingredient is not the drink itself, but the spirit in which it is prepared (we rarely make tea for ourselves in such circumstances) or the goodwill with which it is served? One of life's little imponderables not without irony in the current circumstances given that this cup of comfort contained caffeine which, taken in excess, exacerbates some of the symptoms causing my admission.

Once the tea had worked its way through the system, I was desperate for a wee. No easy undertaking when it entailed being chaperoned by various monitors and applicators to which I remained connected. Rather than make a dive for it, I caught the eye of a staff nurse who firmly instructed me to stay put. Apparently, I was in no fit state to be perambulating around the ward unassisted and would need to 'tie a knot in it' until alternative arrangements could be put in place.

In the period that followed, I began to regret imbibing a second cup. To my considerable relief, just as my bladder was about to explode, a young man attired in yet another shade of blue arrived carrying a cardboard carafe resembling a misshapen vase with its neck set to one side. He drew the curtains around my bed and handed over the container like a baton in a relay race before beating a hasty retreat. This is a strange looking toilet, I mused, and soon discovered there was an art to its use requiring a steady hand, an eye for angles and an ear for discerning when the plimsoll line had been reached. With time (and much practice), I came to recognise the importance of performing these little tasks solo. It was one of the very few ways in which I could preserve a measure of dignity and self-respect.

A green-coated porter was my next caller, announcing relocation. Once unmoored from my anchorage, we embarked on a precarious voyage requiring considerable dexterity as my pilot navigated around obstacles, through the narrow doorway of the ward entrance and along a heavily trafficked corridor before running the gauntlet past the clashing jaws of an elevator. En route, I was struck by the seemingly endless flow of human beings. Some were striding out purposefully whilst others were faltering and seemed lost. There were couples holding hands, parents 'shushing' their children, doctors consulting their pagers, domestics mopping the floor, nurses escorting the sick, electricians changing light fittings, administrators laden with files and a conscientious middle-aged man sanitising his hands at one of those wall-mounted dispensers. I noticed patients heading for the theatre and others skulking off for a smoke. There were visitors, bearing grapes and flowers, eager for reunion with their loved ones, and tearful souls with forlorn faces who looked as if they had just bade farewell to theirs. Various languages travelled the airways celebrating a rich diversity of culture and creed. My nostrils filled with a miasma of fragrance, disinfectant and sweat. It felt as if we were passing through a microcosm of the human race. I marvelled at how we managed to occupy the same space without falling over one another – finding a measure of peace in a common pursuit of healing, temporarily transcending our differences.

My harbour for the night was a six-bed bay within the *Acute Referral Unit* or *ARU* for the uninitiated. Once we had docked at the second berth on the right, a dark blue uniform approached purposefully. It was Matron. Her commanding presence silenced conversation and secured attention in a similar manner to a headmistress descending upon a disorderly class. Even the bugs stopped infecting! She consulted my *Book of Life* before informing me that further tests were necessary before diagnosis would be possible. I wanted to know more but felt too breathless to ask. Instead, I pulled one of those resigned, semi-appreciative expressions and nodded.

Hot on her heels was a rather less formidable member of staff carrying a small tray. "I've come to take some blood," she announced, before lining up half a dozen vials on the top of my bedside locker, like soldiers on parade. I wanted to inquire exactly how much blood "some" was, but thought better of it. After all, she was only trying to help – a judgement that would soon be sorely tested. An elastic tourniquet was applied to my upper right arm causing the vessels to protrude. "There's a nice one," she enthused, before attempting to spear it with a needle. Her first prick was unsuccessful as was the second and third. I wondered whether my veins were armour-plated. Or was the needle blunt? Or should I volunteer my spectacles?

By the time we shifted to the left arm, the atmosphere was charged, frenetic. Stakes had been raised and reputations were on the line. The next lunge felt more like prospecting for any vein willing to oblige than targeting one in particular. The accompanying pain, which at the outset was no more than an uncomfortable pinprick, had become little short of excruciating. I would have readily divulged intimate state secrets or confessed to the most heinous crime to stop it. Now I felt under the spotlight – was my threshold so low that I couldn't tolerate the odd prod without wincing and whining? At least it was distracting me from other concerns. Then, with a stroke of good fortune, success. The soldiers received their rations and all was well.

Blood tests would become a regular feature in the coming weeks as my inner arms took on a freckled complexion born of repeated piercing. It is remarkable how the same procedure can be undertaken in so many different ways and with such varying degrees of success. There is also a fascinating hierarchy that comes into play when dealing with problematic patients. Although clearly visible, the thread-like quality of my veins apparently renders them difficult to puncture. Blood extraction, deemed a relatively straightforward procedure, is often undertaken by relatively junior members of staff. However, whilst technically uncomplicated, it requires considerable skill and a lot of practice to perfect. What tends to happen in tricky cases such as mine is that senior members are drafted in who, having lost the edge owing to lack of practice, miss the mark as often as hit it. Believe me, when it comes to phlebotomy, take your chances with a trainee nurse boasting plenty of active service over a Registrar in the reserves. Heart transplants – well, that's another matter!

The final excursion for the evening was to the X-ray department. By now it was late, yet to my amazement things were still in full swing. Unlike the Almighty who purportedly takes a break on the Sabbath, many NHS services now operate 24/7. After a short wait, I was wheeled into a treatment room, asked to stand motionless and given detailed instructions about posture. I have never quite understood why it is deemed necessary to adopt such contorted positions when posing for X-rays. "Head up, chest out, shoulders back, arms behind with palms up-facing. Now take a deep breath and hold it!" At that point the radiographer retreated to a lead-lined bunker before pressing the mushroom-shaped button. Then a loud click followed by silence. Breathing a sigh of relief, I relaxed the half Nelsons only to be informed that I had moved and would need to repeat the entire rigmarole. Who says modelling is easy?

Chapter 4

Waiting, Waiting, Waiting (*Interlude*)

Although a diagnosis would not be forthcoming until morning, reconnection to the heart monitor once back in *ARU* confirmed something needed to be done before then to reduce the pulse rate and stabilise the heart rhythm. The duty Registrar was summoned. Then followed a prolonged period of waiting. Waiting, if you think about it, is what patients do: waiting upon the disease, waiting to be diagnosed, waiting to be treated, waiting for the treatment to work, waiting to recover, waiting upon carers, waiting for visitors to arrive, waiting for (some) visitors to depart. So much waiting! As I looked around, the bay took on the semblance of a well-equipped waiting room with beds on which patient-waiters were expected to wait patiently.

I've never been much good at waiting. It seemed such a waste of time. Much better to be busy and productive – to be doing something worthwhile. After all, waiting is the prerogative of the incapable or the indolent and I was neither. But all this was about to change as, sentenced to wait, I was forced to rethink.

There are many kinds of waiting: waiting to catch a bus, waiting for a seed to germinate, waiting for the birth of a child, waiting for the death of a loved one, waiting for news, waiting for results, waiting for someone to arrive, waiting to fall asleep, waiting for sunrise, waiting for the whistle at full-time, waiting at a supermarket checkout, waiting for the post, waiting to fall in love, waiting for retirement, waiting for supper, waiting for the end of a working day, waiting to go on holiday, waiting to recover, yes, even waiting to die.

It dawned on me that waiting as a way of being is not without value. In fact, it can be liberating in an odd sort of way. I came to think of it as a gift of time to yourself – space eked out from the demands, preoccupations and routines of existence which is yours to spend as you choose. To make the most of it, though, you need to park those things you 'should' be doing in the knowledge that they are in good hands or will be waiting (there's that word again) for you when you are ready to pick them up once more.

This is not as easy as it sounds. It was long after being discharged from hospital that I managed to lay to rest the ghost of unfulfilled expectations, and weeks later to gain the upper hand over the attendant guilt and worry. What makes this so difficult is that many of us are programmed to be productive. We need to be busy and draw much of our sense of self-worth from what we accomplish as well as from the network of relationships associated with our employments. More than that, our identity as persons becomes determined by the roles we fulfil. Hardly surprising, then, that waiting can seem unnatural and alien.

Personally, it was only by struggling on with tasks and duties until hitting a brick wall that I found a measure of freedom to start waiting creatively. Then, beginning to explore this opportunity, I soon encountered a host of distractions. An obvious candidate is self-preoccupation. With time on our hands and the noise of busy lives subdued, we become more aware of ourselves and our ailments. This, in turn, can spawn an increased sensitivity to our bodily functions where even the slightest change in condition is amplified out of all proportion. For instance, monitoring pulse and blood pressure became almost an obsession. With my own apparatus at home, I could chart their ebb and flow to my heart's content or, as it happened, discontent – every reading supplying grounds for reassurance or panic.

Another distraction is the Internet, especially feeding your ailments into a search engine and following up on the hits. This is not to be recommended unless you possess a strong constitution. The point to remember with the *World Wide Web* is that it is indiscriminate, which means you are as likely as not to land on a site designed for the eyes of medical professionals where the patient-friendliness filter has been removed. I recall happening upon one that went into graphic detail about various treatment options and associated complications for my condition as well as its impact on prognosis and life expectancy. Sometimes you can be confronted with just too much reality.

TV, radio, multimedia, music and audiobooks are other alternatives readily available to patients with time on their hands. And illness can be so overwhelming that sometimes we simply lack the capacity to do anything beyond surviving each moment or allowing ourselves to become lost within distractions able to rescue us from restlessness, pain or despair. For all that, though, there is much to be said for aiming to take responsibility for our waiting rather than becoming casualties of it.

This requires patience and forbearance which are always worth cultivating. It starts with planting our *waiting gardens* purposefully and with care. There are all sorts of seeds available depending on the size of plot, the nature of our condition and, of course, our inclination and preferences. *Appreciating* is a good place to start. Rather than fixating on what we cannot do, focus on what we can. In this respect, hospitals are effective forcing sheds because we inevitably bump into people worse off than ourselves. Without wishing to derive comfort from misfortune, sometimes it is only through exposure to the plight of others that we are able to gain perspective on our own situation. I found appreciating a sure way of holding on to the giftedness of life when all else seemed barren and bleak. And it's infectious. Before long, I was appreciating not only the measure of health I enjoyed, but also the benefits of the NHS, the care of loved ones, those little graces we readily take for granted – even lukewarm tea. And others can catch it too. After all, being miserable isn't part of the patients' charter!

Consideration is a hardy perennial suitable for most terrains. When we come to think of it, for much of life we tend to use one another in a consensual sort of way. We relate *functionally* in terms of what you can do for me or I can do for you rather than *personally* where we recognise each other as human beings. Life would be impossible if we didn't. For instance, I expect the Registrar (thinking back to *ARU*) to relate to me as a medical professional rather than as someone who has recently divorced or purchased a new house or is looking forward to going on holiday. Yet all of these are part of her story. By acknowledging that each of us is so much more than the roles we play, we gain a deeper sense of, and respect for, one another. This can be a hugely rewarding exercise enabling us to grow in empathy, understanding and appreciation. It can even liberate us to be generous in the midst of adversity. As a patient, I found this a blessing. Here was something I could give, even when feeling useless – a word of thanks, a welcoming smile, an affirming note, a prayer offered, a hope expressed. The undeclared sacraments of human encounter.

Reflection, no doubt, is the name of a genetically-modified rose with a subtle pale complexion and a scent reminiscent of an air freshener. But its namesake is ideally suited to the conditions of our gardens in waiting. It comes in many varieties. For instance, there is *Reflecto Retrospectum* (retrospection) where we take stock. This can be rather more far-reaching than sifting through the contents of our short-term memories like an enthu- siastic prospector at a car boot sale. It resembles pilgrims pausing at a cairn to look back over the terrain covered to date as they become conscious of where they have reached on their journeys. This sounds rather demanding when we are already feeling below par. But this is our opportunity and it may not come our way again. Under normal circumstances the pace of life is just too frenetic or, alternatively, we have developed strategies to divert our attention elsewhere. Illness forces us to wait. Let us learn to make the most of it.

In the coming days, I found myself revisiting why it was that my heart had decided to go AWOL when it did. Was it genetically programmed to do so? Had I contracted some condition by chance or caused it by something I had done? Was the body complaining about my propensity to overwork or some other aspect of my lifestyle? I did not particularly want to engage with these questions, but recognised the importance of doing so. Suffering the condition was debilitating enough without being victimised by it also. And this was my way of breaking free from the latter by retracing my footsteps to discover how it was they had led me to this point.

Reflecto Existentialum (attention) is another productive strain. It may seem a strange thing to say, but we spend very little time occupying *now*. We are rarely present in the present. Most of the time our minds are elsewhere. We are thinking about what we have just done or where we are about to go or what our loved ones are doing or whether to apply for a job or what to cook for tea or where to go on holiday or whom we would rather be with or how to fix the kettle that exploded when we forgot to fill it with water because of daydreaming! We are so busy reflecting on the past or anticipating the future that we have no time to occupy the present.

If you don't believe me, recall some of your recent conversations. How much listening and responding was going on, rather than talking at or past one another? How often do our 'conversations' consist of two monologues delivered concurrently with minimal interaction? Or what about a friend of ours who, whenever we meet up, spends most of the time arranging the next get-together instead of making the most of this one.

As we begin to abide in the present, to occupy it wholeheartedly and for its own sake, then not only do we become much more aware of our surroundings, but all sorts of things begin to surface from within: How am I? Who am I? Where am I? What really matters? How is life shaping up? Am I 'on course'? Who sets the compass? But surely, I hear you say, illness is the worst possible state in which to attempt this. After all, here is a present from which we wish to be absent. This is an entirely reasonable response, but it overlooks one of life's greatest challenges, namely to occupy the present moment without being overwhelmed by it – to find space to be present and undiminished even when everything around us seems unpleasant and threatening. Being ill is as good a time to take this on as any.

And, finally, *Reflecto Anticipatum* (anticipation). Unsurprisingly, we instinctively find ourselves conceiving all sorts of scenarios when grounded by illness. That first evening, my mind was spinning with various diagnoses and their implications. What about my nearest and dearest – were they alright, how would this affect them, were they being cared for? Who would cover my bases and undertake those family tasks that fall to me? Then there was work – how was all this going to impact on my job, would I need to take time off, what repercussions would it have upon my colleagues and students, would I be able to catch up?

Although inconceivable during those first few intense hours of crisis, I would soon discover that life goes on. Families pull together and compensate, colleagues rally round and provide cover, clients are reasonable and adjust (mostly), deadlines are revised, some parties even flourish among the new opportunities, challenges and responsibilities someone's incapacity inadvertently spawns. It seems that whilst illness visits ill fortune on the sufferer it can bring the best out in others as they tap into those rich seams of our humanity, resourcing us to be generous and compassionate beyond self-interest.

This last observation is both reassuring and threatening. I felt relief on realising that, functionally speaking, the business usually filling my days was being looked after by others. However, with this came the uncomfortable realisation of my own dispensability. I was not essential. I could be replaced! This is a disquieting recognition on a number of counts, not least because most of us need to be needed. We possess an innate yearning to be valued and significant – one that readily convinces us we have a unique and irreplaceable contribution to make. But for the most part we don't, and to acknowledge as much hurts. It feels diminishing at a time when illness has already impoverished us. Yet, disillusionment of this kind, painful as it is, can yield a more authentic sense of self. It can also release those sharing our lives from any web of dependency we may have woven around them.

It would be disingenuous to leave things there. For personal identity and worth cannot be equated with our output or productivity. In truth, these are expressions, rather than definitions, of our personhood. It is to relationships we should turn when seeking the core of our being and the particular contribution each of us makes. We will have occasion to explore this later; here, let me simply sow another seed, namely to propose that above all it is our relationships which make us who we are and where our particular contribution as persons resides. For instance, any suitably qualified professional could fill my shoes at work, but there is an irreplaceable (for good or ill) dimension to the collegiality shared when I am present. Equally (and here I had better tread carefully), my wife could have married someone else and found fulfilment in that person's companionship, but her experience of marriage and its contribution to her growth as a person would inevitably have been different.

If you think about it, there is a personal component to almost all of our relationships: partners and children, parents and siblings, colleagues, neighbours and friends, teachers and clergy, doctors and dentists, the window cleaner, shop assistant and refuse collector, even the plumber, electrician or tax adviser. In each case, there is a personal dimension to our interactions which extends beyond the purely transactional and draws us into encounter. Here, 'who we are' rather than 'what we do' is the distinguishing feature and characterises our particular contribution to the relationship. From this perspective, it is perhaps helpful to think of our impact on others as concentric ripples emanating from an epicentre where those closest to us feel our absence more keenly than those further away.

There is another aspect of *Reflecto Anticipatum* when illness ceases to be an unwelcome intruder who has broken into our days and becomes instead a signpost on our journey through life. Road signs come in various shapes, sizes and colours depending on their message. Some warn of forthcoming hazards, others of changes in direction or speed limit, others still of approaching junctions. The art of safe driving is learning to interpret the signs aright. What kind of signpost was my illness? In the coming weeks, I found it to be a combination of all three – a hazard warning leading to decisions that would dramatically change the course of my life. But let's not jump the gun.

Waiting, then, as I hope this chapter affirms, was one of my surprise discoveries as a patient. At the outset, it felt arid and barren. It became a fruitful place. The transition was far from quick or painless. I wouldn't have chosen to make it nor can I take any credit for having done so. Perhaps, waiting is itself a grace.

One further blessing waiting bestowed was a *heightened sensory awareness*. It seems incongruous to maintain that sensing takes time, but actually it does, which may explain why I was such an impatient listener. Illness created space for the senses. I found myself sensing with a depth of attention and empathy I had rarely experienced. Although my hearing is mediocre at best, I was able to tune in to the texture of silence, the moods of birdsong, the melody of the breeze, the timbre of voices, the overture of a boiling kettle, the language of bees, the monologues of trees, the coursing of blood though the ears and the bass thud of the beating heart resounding deep within the bowels.

There was time to look beyond those snapshots of the world we make do with and to receive a visual impression of that which awaits us before our eyes. Walks with Tess were sometimes little short of transfigurations as nature became present in its variegated glory. One outing on a crispy winter's morning yielded the following lines:

Below zero...
water sticks to tarmac
and lazy streams slow and stop
to contemplate the moment;
toasty leaves crick and crackle,
and muddy paths refuse to yield
to strides of advancing feet;
fields wear a pale complexion
powdered with icy confection,
sparkling in ambient light;
barren trees bear their bows
dancing in the whimsical winds,
naked save for an arid beauty;
barn doors reveal their batons
and snowflakes hang out to dry
upon threads carrying our voices;
and rabbits scamper to and fro
frolicking in the frosty residues
before diving beneath the earth.
All is held in suspended animation
waiting the dawn
beyond the cusp of a glowing hill.

Did you know you can taste illness? Not just the metallic stain medication deposits on the lips or the acerbic bite of bile gripping the throat, but the staleness of an atrophying body, the blandness of depression, the bitterness of despair. You can also savour the piquant of anticipation, the honeyed butteriness of friendship and the zesty freshness of recovery. You can smell emotions or, at least, sense them in an olfactory way. Fear is pungent and suffo-cating, anxiety is acrid and intoxicating. Joy is that sensation of breathing our fill of clean air whilst happiness is the perfume of a dew-drenched glade on a spring morning. The same goes for touch, which was particularly surprising in my case given that medication had impaired motor coordination and tactile sensi-tivity, but I could still trace the contours of my condition, feel the changing moods of each day and embrace the presence of love in its various embodiments.

I would not be surprised if a wave of incredulity was passing through my readers at this point. And, yes, I would have struggled to believe any of this heightened sensory awareness business as well if it weren't for the fact that circumstances afforded me time to wait upon reality rather than forever demanding reality wait upon me.

Enough waiting, let's return to that first night in *ARU*.

Chapter 5

The First Night

It took me a few moments to realise that the plain-clothed person consulting my *Book of Life* was the long-awaited Registrar. In stark contrast to uniformed members of staff, hospital doctors tend to wear mufti, with a NHS ID badge the only clue to their professional credentials. The other veil over her identity was youthfulness – she just didn't look old enough! Mind you, there can be few surer measures of your progression through the Shakespearean 'ages of man' than protesting how doctors, teachers and bank managers look as if they're barely out of nappies. Be that as it may, after consulting my notes, observing the monitors and wielding her stethoscope with skilful aplomb, I was written up for beta-blockers and digitalis.

To be frank, ingesting neither of these drugs was an appetising prospect. My only experience of the former was during treatment for that ectopic heartbeat back in the 1980s when paralysis was induced rendering me incapable of walking, swallowing or speaking. Digitalis, on the other hand, conjured up images from an Agatha Christie novel or of James Bond collapsing after downing a spiked cocktail during a high-stakes poker game in *Casino Royale*. But my predicament required urgent intervention, so apprehension was relegated to the recesses of my mind. Trust beckoned once more.

'Poisons' safely consumed, it was time to settle down for the night. At least that is what I had been encouraged to do yet, for reasons anyone who has ever been an inpatient will know only too well, is all but impossible to achieve. For one thing, especially at the beginning, everything is strange and unpredictable – the surroundings, personnel, routines, treatments and expectations are unknown quantities. Anxiety abounds, which is why those 'little graces' of human encounter alluded to previously offer a lifeline.

What I needed in those first fraught hours of hospitalisation extended beyond the expertise of medical professionals and the active ingredients of medication. I needed reassurance that I wasn't alone – that my current predicament hadn't put me beyond the reach of personal warmth and kindness, that those accompanying me through these uncertain times were not clinical automatons with faces, but fellow human beings with hearts. When searching for signs of life, even the slightest intimation of empathy or goodwill dispenses a wholly disproportionate dose of therapeutic benefit. A truth expressed so memorably in a short poem, entitled *Saving Grace*:

Fish do not smile, nor birds: their faces are not
Equipped for it. A smiling dog's the illusion
And wish-fulfilment of its owner. Cats wear
Permanent smiles inspired by mere politeness.
But human animals at times forget their
Godlike responsibilities; the tension
Slackens, the weasel-sharp intentness falters;
Muscles relax; the eyes refrain from peering
Aside, before and after; and the burden
Of detail drops from forehead; cheekline gently
Creases; the mouth wide-flowers; the stiff mask softens;
And Man bestows his simple, unambitious,
Unservile, unselfseeking, undeceptive,
Uncorrupt gift, the grace-note of a smile.
– ASJ Tessimond, 1902–62

What is more, we inevitability become preoccupied with the condition that caused our admission in the first place. Whether suffering symptoms, managing treatment, anticipating prognosis or contemplating the impact on others, every waking moment is sucked into an ever-expanding vortex of dis-ease. That first night, I was transfixed by the apparatus monitoring my heart, watching the ebb and flow of its vital statistics like a city analyst scrutinising the stock market. Whilst blood pressure remained consistently 'bearish', my pulse resembled the 'boom and bust' of the 80s and 90s. One minute it would be pushing 180 before diving to 60, 50 or even 40 beats per minute. It was an object lesson in helplessness – all I could do was look on with the racked attention of an investor whose livelihood was in the balance. Even those sparse moments of relief dozing-off affords were abruptly curtailed by an alarm sounding each time a hazardously high or low reading was registered. Not the gentlest of wake-up calls.

Then there is the self-evident observation that, in a hospital ward, you aren't alone. The side-bay of six beds in which I had been placed was full. I was flanked by middle-aged men recovering from the effects of hypoglycaemia. On the other side to the left was a young woman suffering from an overdose. The far right berth was occupied by a fractious character recovering from emergency surgery performed on some part of his digestive tract. However, rather than relaxing into convalescence, his outlook was that of a prisoner seeking parole whilst arranging an escape should his overtures prove unsuccessful. Petitioning for early release, phoning home to confirm the getaway car was on standby and checking his knapsack contained essentials continued throughout the night until, discerning a window of opportunity, he made a break for it dressed in little more than one of those endearing green theatre gowns and a pair of bedroom slippers, much to the bemusement of the nursing staff and relief of the rest of us.

Immediately opposite me was an elderly woman who must have been ninety, if a day. To her, at least, sleep was second nature. That is pretty much all she did apart from stir when bidden to take medication or at the sound of an approaching meals trolley – evidently, there was nothing ailing with her appetite! It was her heart rate, though, that caught my attention. It made mine look positively pedestrian. In fact, I wondered whether her monitor was on the blink given the scale and speed of fluctuation. To find a suitable analogy, we must leave the 'square mile' and head for the fairground. Her pulse rate, peaking in the high 100s before plunging into the depths only to bounce back and then repeat the cycle over and over again, resembled the crests and troughs of a roller coaster. Yet, through it all, she appeared oblivious to her runaway heart and surprisingly unaffected by its antics.

Although I had often heard stories about the banter between inpatients finding solidarity in their circumstances, thrown together by a twist of fate, the communication between the six of us was sparse and perfunctory. Like castaways shipwrecked on discrete islands within shouting distance, we respected each other's domain whilst keeping a close eye on the comings and goings of adjacent colonies. During that first night, there were few verbal exchanges; instead, communication was conducted through the cacophony of automated alarms emanating from our monitors each time some bodily function transgressed the register of normal operation.

I found a measure of distraction in the nocturnal habits of my bedfellows, reflecting on how exposed we become when sleep incapacitates, especially when we're being observed:

Sneezing, snoring, grinding of teeth,
wincing, writhing and blows,
talking whilst sleeping,
walking whilst keeping
one's legs beneath the bed clothes.
Trips to the toilet and cries out for help,
belching whilst picking one's nose,
internal combustion,

external disruption
once someone's delivered a commode.

Another reason why sleep can be so elusive is the activities of the night shift as members go about their duties. I was surprised at just how much takes place during those curfew hours. Tasks extended far beyond mounting a watching brief and reacting to the necessities of the moment: distributing medication, taking temperatures and BPs, updating records, prepping syringe drivers, changing infusion bags, measuring urine output, checking insulin levels to name but a few. Then, whenever a berth was vacated (in our case, following the 'great escape'), a thorough cleansing ensued with everything from the oxygen mask to the locker interior receiving a liberal dose of disinfectant or being replaced altogether. Then, no sooner was one name erased from the whiteboard above the bed than another took its place as, mattress still warm and the scent of alcohol spray hanging in the air, the next inhabitant was transported to his or her island retreat.

The rate of throughput in a busy NHS facility needs to be witnessed to be believed. In certain respects, acute hospitals resemble vast automotive accident and repair shops, in this case for mending bodies that weren't assembled very well in the first place or have been damaged through the passage of time or are simply wearing out. They also handle deliveries, disposals and MOTs. Each 'vehicle' passes through the diagnostic bay, on site or in local branches, before being transferred to the appropriate department for specialised attention from whence they are released for further tours of trouble-free motoring (at least, that's the goal).

I recognise this is a rather mechanistic way of looking at things, but it affords some insight to the scale and complexity of the enterprise. Quite naturally, when 'in the system', we think it is all there for us and become critical, even indignant, when there are delays or things fail to go according to plan. In one sense, hospitals do exist for you and me, but there are a lot of us and we don't always take our turn in becoming ill or, for that matter, keep our illnesses to ourselves when we do. Nor should we overlook that in any hospital there are far more members of staff than patients, each experiencing their own life issues and challenges. Then, factor in how, for all their expertise, doctors are still honing their skills, experimenting with new treatments, pioneering procedures etcetera and it's a miracle so many of us emerge a good deal healthier than when we entered.

There is something awesome here. That first night, I was struck by the sheer scale of it all and deeply appreciative that as a society we hadn't shied away from attempting to implement such a thoroughgoing humanitarian vision – free health care for all at the point of need. Of course, it is far from perfect (although I am not sure what 'perfect' would mean in this context), but it is infinitely preferable to what awaits the majority of the global population should they happen to fall ill. I felt an uneasy connectedness with the rest of the human race. Whilst, to a member, we are bound together by a 'sickness unto death' from which not even the healthiest are immune, some of us, through accidents of birth, have access to comprehensive health care provision whilst others suffer and die from some of the most easily treatable of conditions. It was a disturbing realisation, tinged with guilt and sadness, causing me to confront the injustice of privilege and the responsibilities visited upon its beneficiaries.

The all-embracing scope of illness and the enormity of the challenge of responding to the suffering it engenders highlights one of the dilemmas facing healthcare providers, namely how to deliver a service that is all-inclusive yet capable of responding to human need personally and individually. No doubt, millions of people around the world are affected by the same complaint as me and we would all benefit from the best research and treatment programmes. Yet each of us is so much more than the condition. Our well-being is determined by a complex web of interactions and conditions which cannot be satisfactorily restored or maintained by medical treatment alone. We need to be related to as persons. And how difficult that must be for healthcare professionals who are attending to the sick and the dying every day of their working lives.

Such thoughts and reflections, interspersed with bouts of heart monitoring, patient watching and anxiety, were my companions during that first vigil. The night passed so slowly that no second went unnoticed. I can remember few occasions when the present claimed so much of my attention and I can think of few times when I so longed to escape my circumstances and be somewhere else. If the passing of time was measured by the impact of intense experience upon our lives, my birthday count must have advanced by leaps and bounds.

Finally, a nurse tipped the light switch, causing fluorescent tubes to burst into life, before advancing on the window curtains with unfettered strides announcing the arrival of another day. Soon afterwards the well-oiled wheels of the breakfast trolley could be heard approaching, laden with ample supplies of those essential medicines – tea and toast!

Chapter 6

Ward Round

The first few hours of the new day were busy with routine. Cleaning was high on the agenda, undertaken by various uniforms – the blues and the greens, the browns and the whites – each with their designated duties. Patients were invited to remove the stale sweat of a sticky night. Depending on one's condition this ranged from full-immersion to a much more modest affair. Mine fell into the latter category owing to various attachments anchoring me to the bedside. A towel and bowl of warm water were supplied and the curtains delimiting my island habitat drawn. The rest was up to me.

It is surprising what can be accomplished with a relatively small quantity of H_2O. I remember reading as a child of how Bedouins were able to carry out their daily toileting, including brushing their teeth, in no more than a mug full of water. Although, by contrast, I was positively swimming in the stuff, washing your armpits and nether regions without pulling out cannulas or disconnecting monitors requires a good deal more ingenuity than I was accustomed to investing in such mundane tasks. Be that as it may, I made a fist of it discovering en route what Arab desert-dwellers know only too well, namely the importance of performing one's ablutions in the right order.

That first morning wash proved to be revealing in all sorts of ways. For one thing, it caused me to acknowledge a side effect of illness I had not anticipated and would struggle to accommodate: the amount of time and energy expended on those everyday activities that hitherto passed unnoticed. I was reminded of that slightly risqué definition of advancing years, "When it takes all night to do what you used to do all night." Being a patient has its equivalent. Previously, I had given little thought to the rudimentary operations of subsistence, most of which relate to our bodies in one way or another – feeding, cleaning, disposing of waste products. They all seemed very much 'second division', to be fitted in around premier league fixtures. Suddenly, they had been promoted.

The ancient Celtic way of life, still preserved and practised in parts of Scotland, bears witness to a rich seam of spirituality rooted in ordinary experience where you can find a prayer to accompany almost every daily task. Here's one for facial ablutions which, as it happens, resonates with the words of blessing pronounced at Christian baptism:

> *The palmful of the God of Life*
> *The palmful of the Christ of Love*
> *The palmful of the Spirit of Peace,*
> *Triune*
> *Of grace.*
> *– Carmina Gadelica*

You may or may not be the praying kind and, even those of us who are, may struggle with this form of words. Yet, I suspect it expresses an aspiration we can all relate to – the hallowing of the ordinary, the imbuing of the essential material of existence with meaning and significance. When struggling with ill health, a disproportionately high percentage of waking life is taken up with that category of activities we would normally never mention if someone asked us how we had spent our day. Now these incidentals make up our day and the challenge is to find value within their execution.

> *I never thought that life could get this small,*
> *that I would care so much about a cup,*
> *the taste of tea, the texture of a shawl,*
> *and whether or not I should get up.*

I'm not unhappy. I have learnt to drift
and sip. The smallest things are gifts.
– From *Chemotherapy* by Julia Darling

Establishing routine has a vital contribution to make here. After all, there can be few things more threatening than oceans of featureless time – days bereft of structure or content where there is nothing to anticipate or engage in, nothing to occupy our hands, hearts and minds. Hospitals, like many institutions, are the complete antithesis to this. They are animated by routine from the instant the automated doors open to admit us to the moment they close behind our backs, returning us to the outside world. Although such imposition of order may initially seem alien and threatening, as patients and staff are required to conform to prescribed patterns of behaviour, there is reassurance in the predictability it affords and confidence in the expectation we will be cared for according to professionally recognised standards. Paradoxically, although the prospect of the next scheduled injection or visit from the physiotherapist may fill us with dread, such activities can be cairns upon our journey through the next twenty-four hours and, in a way, serve as stepping stones towards recovery. In the coming days, before and after discharge, I would come to appreciate the importance of routines – the rhythms of the day, as I like to call them – which are no less essential for wholesome living than the healthy beating of a human heart. But I digress.

Once we had all been topped and tailed, beds straightened, floors cleaned, surfaces dusted and water jugs recharged, the rainbow of uniforms slowly faded. We were left waiting once more. Ten-thirty was too early for lunch (even within a hospital time zone) and visitors were not expected until afternoon. The sound of an approaching tea trolley was no more than wishful thinking. Yet you could taste the sense of anticipation tinged with apprehension, insecurity and equivocation. The atmosphere was subdued with the six of us lost in our own thoughts. Conversation was sparse and stilted, restricted to the perfunctory and conducted between persons whose attention lay elsewhere.

What or who was the cause of this change in climate? Everybody seemed to know but me and, for some reason, I couldn't muster the courage to ask. This time, ignorance seemed preferable to interrupting the singular focus pervading the present moment and demonstrating my naivety to the institutionalised world now defining my existence. Thankfully, before the suspense reached fever pitch, the answer emerged.

It began with muffled voices, then the sound of an approaching flotilla. Finally, it arrived – the Consultant with his team. To my great relief, they docked at another bed, the first on the left nearest the entrance, which, assuming linear progression, put me as the fifth port of call. Plenty of time to observe, I thought. The Consultant wore a similar youthfulness to the duty Registrar of the previous night. His 'uniform' was stethoscope and ID badge; no white coat or green surgical pyjamas. He was accompanied by half a dozen supporters comprising medical students, hospital doctors and 'she who must be obeyed' (incidentally, what is the term for a collection of medics – a dose of doctors, a prescription of pharmacists, a bandage of nurses, a transfusion of haematologists, an arsenic of anaesthetists?). Each patient was surrounded by this entourage before the bedside curtains were drawn around them with exemplary precision, affording a measure of privacy. In truth, it was a token gesture. Printed cotton is not renowned for its soundproofing qualities which enabled the entire ward to be privy to what was going on within this makeshift consulting room. And, despite pretending otherwise, we all listened intently, hanging on every detail, eager to learn the fate of our island neighbours. On more than one occasion, I had to check myself from proffering an unsolicited opinion or observation.

There is something ironic, even perverse, about this. We are in hospital because of illness which, of itself, signals a loss of independence and self-determination. Then, our vulnerability is intensified through being subjected to the dispassionate gaze of medics and their apprentices together with the flapping ears of hospital bedfellows, most of whom hadn't heard of the Hippocratic Oath never mind being bound by it. As a priest, I often had members of the parish coming round for a chat during which they would share the most sensitive of intimacies, confident the 'seal of confession' ensured nothing would pass beyond those four walls. But here the walls were permeable, with details of our case history and medical condition passing unfiltered into the public domain. I wondered how the Consultant and his team would feel about the appropriateness of these arrangements if roles were reversed. Then another thought crossed my mind: does vulnerability have a part to play within the dynamics of healing? Perhaps such impotence and exposure engender a trusting openness and heightened receptivity which relate us to sources of wholeness and well-being beyond ourselves or, alternatively, energise those capacities integral to our own personhood.

Eventually, it was my turn in what, by then, had become a familiar routine. The fabric walls enveloped us, creating a cosy, almost claustrophobic, atmosphere. Matron offered a brief medical résumé before outlining the current treatment plan. The Consultant, having familiarised himself with my *Book of Life* and conducted a superficial anatomical examination whilst asking various questions about presenting symptoms, previous bouts of ill health and general lifestyle, turned to his colleagues and addressed them as if I wasn't there. The subsequent exchange deepened my sense of powerlessness – it was a conversation about me, or at least a specimen of *homo sapiens* exhibiting symptoms identical to my own, from which I had been excluded not by being absent but through being ignored. I tried to listen in as I had done for the patients before me – eavesdropping on my own consultation.

Once concluded, the Consultant turned to me again before passing judgement. At least, that's how it felt. Having weighed the evidence, the jury of experts withdrew for deliberation before reaching a verdict which was subsequently delivered to the accused. It came upon me as an imposition rather than as an interpretation. The distinction is more than semantic reflecting a confrontational, moralising approach – them and me, professionals and patient, powerful and impotent – where the illness was viewed as a bodily misdemeanour to be punished and eradicated. This left me with a strong sense that my heart was not simply malfunctioning, but had done something wrong!

This did little to enhance the patient-practitioner rapport or to establish trust between us. As a concession, I was given leave to appeal. "Any questions?" There followed another moment of eloquent speechlessness. Should I apologise for the fickleness of my frame and for allowing myself to become ill? Or should I protest my innocence and defend the accidental nature of my condition? And what of ameliorating circumstances – after all, I was a hard-working public servant who spent most of his waking life ministering to the needs of others. I paid my taxes and was a law-abiding citizen. In the end, I remained silent and awaited the sentencing.

I am aware this sounds critical and in a way it is, but it also highlights two key challenges for anyone working in the caring professions – perhaps, for anyone who dares to care. They both relate to the integrity of persons. That morning, the Consultant was following routine. It was his regular ward round during which he attended to beds full of anonymous people manifesting readily identifiable symptoms and suffering from predictable complaints that required tried and tested courses of treatment or, failing that, were beyond the reach of medical intervention. It was an exercise in professional expertise which presumably was competently undertaken. However, behind each complaint resides a complainant, a patient, a person whose life has been affected, in some cases substantially or terminally, by the reason he or she now occupies a hospital bed. And because illness affects all of life, so the whole person needs to be engaged, responded to and, hopefully, made whole. We are, to use the jargon, psychosomatic beings, a complex web of biological, psychological and spiritual interactions needing to be related to accordingly.

For this reason, like it or not, most of us have an intimate association with illness. Not out of choice (well, not for many of us anyway), but necessity because it is *our* bodies that are diseased. We cannot abstract ourselves from our corporality, like an astronaut shedding a spacesuit, and view our physical frame as an object, an anonymous 'it'. Our bodies not only belong to us, they *are* an integral part of what makes you 'you' and me 'me'. Which means their disease is our disease and how others relate to them, especially those employed to look after them, affects and effects us personally. This is where the 'garage' analogy of the previous chapter proves insightful although inadequate. My bedside consultation had rather too much in common with a competent mechanic investigating a fault on my car.

None of this is new nor is it restricted to the medical profession. After conducting the best part of a thousand funeral services, mainly for persons unknown to me, I am only too familiar with the challenge of ensuring the performance of routine does not become soulless and robotic. Or the way we relate to our fellow humans impersonal and unsympathetic. It was salutary, even if painful and diminishing, to be on the receiving end of an inadvertent object lesson illustrating the point.

When the Consultant's armada upped anchor, I had gained two new letters after my name, AF. Lying in bed, reflecting on my encounter, I had little inkling of how this insignia would change the course of my life. Perhaps it was just as well!

Chapter 7

Naming the Beast

I've never found 'not knowing' easy. Some people seem able to bury themselves in the busyness of the present whilst awaiting important news, but I am not one of them. My mind can think of little else, rehearsing various worse-case scenarios before becoming anxious and apprehensive – the epitome of self-induced paranoia. Total ignorance, when you're blissfully unaware of what you don't know is one thing; but being aware of it, especially when what you know you don't know has serious personal ramifications, is quite another. Such unknowing is potently corrosive, weakening resolve whilst eating away at those foundations providing stability and direction to our lives.

Much better, then, to know. "Naming the beast is halfway to exorcism" is a pearl of wisdom I picked up from one of those self-help manuals on overcoming phobias, although since then I've come to recognise its broader application (regrettably, not extending to a certain person's fear of flying). We need to comprehend the nature and scale of a challenge (or opportunity, for that matter – it's not always bad news) before being able to harness those resources within and beyond which help us to engage constructively and creatively. Without such knowledge, we are at the mercy of our imaginations or somebody else's.

For all that, though, it remains a sobering prospect how many of us host illness without having the slightest inkling. The less debilitating ones come and go, subdued by the body's defences, whilst their more pernicious cousins stalk the back alleys undetected until ready to pounce. During the so-called incubation period, when there are few if any symptoms, we profess to being in fine fettle. We may even visit our GPs for a check-up and receive a clean bill of health. Yet all the while covert forces are conspiring against us. In our ease we are dis-eased. It is only when diagnosed that reality dawns, although as a matter of fact this is the moment of identification not of inception. Before then, we were still suffering from the same medical condition, but the beast had yet to be named!

Come to think of it, much of life takes place within this climate of reality slowly revealing its secrets: a woman finds out she's pregnant, students receiving exam results, pioneers discovering new frontiers, deceit exposed, news of unrequited love, a surprise party. In their own way, each of these discloses something existing before its apprehension. The woman was no less pregnant before the doctor's visit, and the unrequited love no less profound before it was acknowledged. Now delve deeper, beyond the flotsam and jetsam filling our lives, to ponder existence itself. Infirmity beckons us to do no less – to acknowledge that we are not only ill but ILL, suffering from a terminal condition inherited at conception: mortality. Unsurprisingly, most of us try to ignore this diagnosis for as long as possible. Presuming the givenness of today guarantees the prospect of tomorrow, we attend to the preoccupying pastimes of the present whilst striving to make provision for a 'heavenly' retirement. In brief, we live a delusion – immortals in a fleeting world – until reality catches up with us.

At this point, those who've persevered thus far may be tempted to give up, consigning this slim volume to the recycling bin, before its discordant notes ruin the sweet melodies of our days. After all, life is too short to have our noses rubbed in its brevity! Yet I wonder whether Sister Death, as St Francis of Assisi (13th century) described it, has to be viewed in such a negative light, as the archetypal party-pooper. For what is death if not the upper limit to existence, providing shape and definition? Rather than devaluing it, death concentrates life, inviting us to live it for all it is worth. Not to squander a single moment, but to invest our energies in worthwhile pursuits and enduring realities. To discover in each day sufficient joy and meaning to last a lifetime. We have all heard testimonies of those whose brush with death proved to be a passport to life. By reminding us of our mortality, illness beckons us to do likewise.

I don't mean to make light of life's most feared predator. Death is awesome. The prospect overwhelms our minds and profoundly disturbs us at every level. It entails dying which can be prolonged and painful. It requires us to let go of our loved ones as well as much we hold dear and have devoted our time and energy to. I well remember the night in Cambridge during the early 1980s when the inevitability of my own death struck with such force that it flung me into deep depression whilst triggering an aggressive psychosomatic reaction which would take years to understand and manage. During that period, I grieved my own mortality. I suffered its venom and very nearly became its prey. It was one of the most diminishing, yet enriching, periods of my life. A proving process through which much of the superficial clutter we inherit from others or collect en route was burned away, exposing the bare essentials of existence, investing life with fresh impetus and focus. Gradually, I ceased to be death's victim, crushed under the weight of its pall. Now she is my companion, another Franciscan insight, who at some undisclosed point will consume me, but until then encourages me to make the most of each day by living it intentionally, wholeheartedly and with integrity.

I will say more about this process of proving and distillation later, but what I need to emphasise here is that none of this is meant to suggest we adopt a defeatist attitude towards infirmity. "When your number's up there's nothing you can do about it" may hold sway for the National Lottery, but has little to commend it when matters of health are at stake. To the contrary, because life is so precious it shouldn't be squandered or curtailed. We owe it to ourselves, as well as to our loved ones and those who look to us, to take recovery seriously which, to my mind, makes it all but incomprehensible why so many of us seem content to know the beast's name, so to speak, without knowing much about its habits and instincts nor of how it can be overcome.

Years of visiting the sick confirmed my suspicion that the need to understand the nature of our illness or its prognosis is far from widespread. There are those who seem to view bodily repair in a similar light to taking the car to the garage after a breakdown (to return to an analogy deployed last chapter) or to arranging for a builder to call after a storm. You put it in the hands of experts whilst looking to the insurers to cover the cost (in this case the NHS). Such levels of trust may appear laudable, but they are misplaced because the comparison is flawed. We don't own our bodies in the sense of them being a possession like a car or a house. We *are* our bodies and must take ultimate responsibility for their upkeep, maintenance and restoration. This is difficult to accomplish when we are largely ignorant of our medical condition or are not committed to being actively involved in our healing and recuperation.

My beast bears the mark 'AF' or, at least, one of them does – I would discover later there were others even more debilitating. I can remember staring at these initials which the Consultant had inscribed upon my *Book of Life* wondering what they amounted to. A strange diffidence, or was it apprehension, came over me. Did I want to know? Did I *really* want to know? Or should I prolong my ignorance for as long as possible? After all, once the secret was out there was no going back, no way of circumventing its consequences. It was a similar sensation to when, many years previously, I had stood by the telephone in our family home weighing whether to contact school to obtain a set of key examinations results which I suspected would be bad news. After much agonizing, I had done so and my suspicions were confirmed. Before long, the need to know won out on this occasion also.

In contrast to terms such as cancer, coronary thrombosis or cerebral haemorrhage which convey something of the seriousness of the condition to which they refer, Atrial Flutter sounds innocuous and benign, conjuring images of exotic butterflies rather than dangerous predators. But first appearances can be deceptive for AF, together with additional complications and conditions yet to emerge, would prove to be no less flighty and a good deal more menacing. Atrial Flutter is a condition affecting the upper chambers of the heart (the atria) caused by abnormalities in the electrical impulses controlling the contraction of the cardiac muscle. Rather than the natural pacemaker stimulating the atria to fire a charge every second or so, mine had switched into machine gun mode delivering 400 plus rounds per minute in a very unfocused and haphazard manner. As contractions in the atria trigger similar activity in the heart's main pumping chambers, the ventricles, mine were struggling to keep up, hence the tachycardia identified in the ambulance. The net effect is a stressed heart operating inefficiently with its capacity for circulating blood around the body drastically curtailed which left me breathless, lethargic and lightheaded, struggling with chronic fatigue, failing memory and impaired cognitive functioning.

Now the beast was outed, I wanted to know which jungle it had emerged from and why it had preyed on me. These questions instinctively filled my mind in the hours following the ward round. I subsequently learned that AF has many causes. Often it indicates heart disease, high blood pressure or problems with other organs such as an overactive thyroid gland or thrombosis in the lungs. It can be triggered by substances affecting the electrical activity of the heart such as alcohol or caffeine. Stress can be a contributory factor, as can serious infection. Only future tests would reveal the likely provenance of my occurrence. That New Year's Day, however, I found myself cast in the role of a *bon viveur* even though my Hogmanay celebrations amounted to a cup of lukewarm tea and a dry biscuit!

Initially, this seemed little more than a jocular quip, but as the day progressed I sensed we had moved beyond diagnosis rooted in medical science to value judgement based on speculation. A presumption that would subsequently influence how my case was written up and reported. As it happens, further investigations would lead my GP and another Consultant to identify a severe chest infection from which I had been suffering as the most likely cause. But for the rest of my hospital stay, I was a winebibber receiving comeuppance. Suddenly the road to recovery had become steeper – no longer was I simply contending with a malfunctioning heart; now the air had become stifled with moralising eddies. I felt a surge of indignation. Even if the 'Hogmanay hypothesis' had proved well founded, what difference should it make within this context of a NHS hospital? Is the life of a patient suffering from AF brought on by drinking too much inferior in some way or worthy of less medical attention to one where the cause appears morally neutral? In that moment, I experienced a profound empathy with those suffering from the 'pariah' illnesses of our time, as well as for those excluded from treatment on the basis of some other prejudice, ageism a case in point.

Why are we so ready to pigeonhole people according to their illnesses – to evaluate their characters by the nature of their misfortune? The clearest contemporary example must be AIDS where it's assumed infection is a consequence of sexual promiscuity; but there are many others, including lung disease (smoking), obesity (gluttony), drug dependency (profligacy), liver cirrhosis (alcoholism) and chronic fatigue syndrome (indolence/hypochondria). Why is this? Perhaps, because it releases us from any moral obligation we may otherwise feel – a sense of solidarity with those who suffer or responsibility for their well-being, as judgement extinguishes compassion.

Equally striking and no less revealing is how certain medical conditions are more socially acceptable than others. Break your leg playing the 'beautiful game' and you're a hero, but put your back out whilst performing some manoeuvre from the *Kama Sutra* and you're deemed to be a pervert. But it can be more subtle, triggering a heart attack through overwork is a measure of commitment to the cause, whilst courting one through an unhealthy lifestyle is tantamount to treason. And what about our intolerance and lack of understanding of strategies some devise to manage the pressures of expectation or responsibilities of office? "My rule of life prescribed as an absolutely sacred rite: smoking cigars and also the drinking of alcohol before, after and if need be during all meals and in the intervals between them." Somehow, I doubt whether Winston Churchill would have led our nation so effectively through its "darkest hour" fuelled by a diet of cranberry juice and nicotine patches!

Rant over, AF & Co remains. Now to discover how one goes about subduing it.

Chapter 8

The Bitter Pill

There can be few areas of medicine where the word 'practice' is more appropriate than in the prescribing of drugs. I suspect we have all sat on the edge of our seats during one of those TV medic-dramas as the doctor arrives in the nick of time to inject some potent remedy into the bloodstream of a hapless casualty who instantaneously revives. Thankfully, such drugs exist, but so do others that have precisely the opposite effect. What is more, the same preparation can be a miracle cure for one patient and a lethal venom for another. No doubt there are medicines where the therapeutic benefits are universally efficacious, but they are in a minority. In most cases, it's a balance of probability based on clinical tests and previous patterns of usage, with a large margin of error when predicting the impact upon anyone in particular. Basically, when it comes to medication, we're all guinea pigs!

One reason drugs do not always make us better is because diagnosis is partial or incorrect. We may not have been able to describe symptoms with sufficient precision or perhaps they characterise a number of different conditions or belong to a secondary ailment rather than the underlying complaint. Yet, even when correctly diagnosed and prescribed, no two persons respond to medication in the same way. Each of us possesses a unique biochemical profile determining our sensitivity to and tolerance of 'alien' substances which can change through time or in different circumstances. Nor should we overlook the interactions between medicines. This can precipitate catastrophic consequences. Now factor in how effective treatment often extends beyond the active constituents of medicines to include emotional, psychological and sociological factors, and the odds on any of us mounting a recovery begin to lengthen.

Thankfully, most of us do to some measure, but if you think I am exaggerating the problems try reading one of those fact sheets accompanying prescription and, increasingly, over-the-counter drugs – that feat of origami we regularly consign to the waste bin without so much as a cursory glance. Spreading out this tightly-folded leaflet reveals an equally densely-formatted expanse of text explaining the what, who, how and why's of the drug in question. Persevere to the end and you will reach the smallest of 'small print' where principal side effects and interactions are listed. Assuming your eyesight has not failed this can make for sobering reading and, on occasion, will cause you to wonder why anyone would subject their system to such a powerful and unpredictable potion.

This was the situation I found myself in. The following catalogue is lifted from the *Patient Information Leaflet* supplied with the medication I would shortly have little alternative but to commence taking:

> ... weight loss or gain, shortness of breath, coughing, wheezing, changes in heart rate, heart problems or pain in the chest, problems with your vision, restlessness, tiredness, impotence, hair loss, nightmares, sleeplessness, pins-and-needles, dizziness, headaches or fever, incoordination, shaking, numbness, tingling pain, muscle weakness, blue-grey skin colour or skin rashes including tingling, burning, redness, blistering and flaking, inflammation of the testicles, blood disorders, hepatitis, cirrhosis, yellowing of the skin or the whites of the eyes, disturbances in kidney function and inflammation of the blood vessels, nausea, vomiting, or a metallic taste may be noticed.

Believe it or not, these are the edited highlights. Consult a publication prepared for healthcare professionals and you will become acquainted with an even longer list! My leaflet advised that the guidance of a physician should be sought if any of the more serious side effects occurred. Given that death was included in the uncut version, perhaps the services of a funeral director would be more appropriate. Admittedly, the drug in question is notorious. It has spawned user-websites packed with personal testimonies and coping strategies where, no doubt, you can purchase T-shirts imprinted with "I took ********** and survived." Seriously, though, no drug is without its dark side and every cup of life may prove to be for some unfortunate 'exception proving the rule' a poisoned chalice.

In the light of this, providing us patient-consumers (as we have now become) with information on the potential benefits and possible dangers of drugs, medical procedures and the like sound enlightened, affording us the wherewithal to make an informed choice. In many instances, though, this is more apparent than real. If you wake up in the morning with a moderate headache you can choose between aspirin, codeine, ibuprofen, paracetamol, some herbal remedy or even to grin and bear it. But for more serious conditions, the options are drastically reduced, often to little more than whether you take your chances with the symptoms untreated or the side effects of the prescribed remedy.

As I say, this was my predicament. It soon became clear the initial pre-diagnosis drugs were not working. More invasive treatment was ruled out on the short term because of the risk of causing a stroke (one of the principal dangers with Atrial Flutter). The blood would need to be anticoagulated (thinned) before any of these options could be attempted. In the meantime, something had to be done to slow the heart and stabilise the pulse. But what?

The cardiologist I was referred to on returning home to England, together with my GP, recommended a particular drug – the one whose vital statistics are noted above. "What did I think?" I was asked. We rehearsed the arguments for and against. I conducted my own investigations online in an attempt to weigh the evidence in a detached and objective manner. Deepening my dilemma was the recognition that in some cases the drug in question actually exacerbated the symptoms it was prescribed to treat. Rather than equipping me to make an informed choice, exposure to the evidence simply confirmed my sense of power-lessness. In as much as I could think straight about anything, it appeared the least worst option. But, in reality, my decision owed little to critical evaluation and a great deal to trust. It seemed to boil down to the following: Did I trust my medical advisors and was I prepared to entrust my life to their professional judgement? This was the crux. Pushed to the outer reaches of human experience, it was neither the findings of government league tables nor the claims of pharmaceutical companies that proved determinative; instinctively, it was that most essential of human dispositions.

During the process of reaching a conclusion, I was struck by how contrary we can be when interpreting 'odds'. For instance, the chances of winning a fortune at the races or on the *National Lottery* are remote, but we still invest our hard-earned cash when feeling lucky; yet, when it comes to the more extreme side effects of medication, we discount them on the grounds of their rarity! Or again, people who smoke may acknowledge this habit can have a detrimental effect on health, but risk it anyway believing they can run the gauntlet. Each of us, I suspect, has our own Achilles' heel, unprotected by the powers of reason and good sense, where we expose another characteristic of the human spirit, namely a propensity for irrational behaviour and for throwing caution to the wind. I say 'another', although sometimes trust can seem disturbingly similar.

Before the first week of New Year was spent, I had embarked on the AF Diet which was destined to significantly outlast previous Resolutions. It consisted of three special ingredients: a cardiac-specific beta-blocker, an anti-arrhythmia drug and an anticoagulant. Compared to the agonies of cutting back on those delicious, calorie-rich goodies consumed to excess over the festive season, the prospect of swallowing a few multicoloured Smarties didn't strike me as problematic, but I was soon to learn otherwise.

For one thing, the medication needed to be taken at the same time each day, which is straightforward unless your short-term memory is on the blink. This proved to be a real challenge. First, I had to remember to collect the prescriptions from the health centre, then to obtain the drugs from a pharmacy and finally to take them as advised. In practice, though, the situation was more complex because dosage varied through time or was determined by the outcome of blood tests which also had to be remembered as did the revised levels of intake. Furthermore, as my coordination deteriorated, removing tablets from their foil-covered packaging became a nightmare. After repeated attempts, the pill would eventually pop out and hop along the tabletop before plunging to the floor and lodging itself in some inaccessible crevice requiring a further act of extraordinary rendition, during which I would forget what I was about and where I had reached with the daily tablet tally. This seems comical now, but to begin with it was yet further confirmation of my newly acquired status of patient. Thank heavens for diaries, post-it notes and pill boxes.

Another complication was caused by my drugs possessing strange dietary requirements. For instance, the effectiveness of one was greatly reduced when accompanied by too many greens whilst another took exception to grapefruit and cranberries. This was one case where healthy eating was to be avoided at all costs including, as it happens, staples from my daily food intake which, in turn, caused more memory problems. Now I had to remember what *not* to eat.

All this paled into insignificance when the side effects began to kick in. I use the term guardedly because it was often unclear whether something was caused by the underlying condition or its treatment or both. Take memory, as we've already alluded to it. Were my lapses a side effect of the medication or a symptom of the heart not functioning properly? Equally, what about breathlessness, headaches, poor concentration, dizziness, listlessness and chronic fatigue? Others were more readily attributable, although not beyond doubt: dehydration and nausea, muscle weakness, spasm and wasting, nightmares, hallucinations and disrupted sleep, skin dryness, discolouration and blistering, blurred vision, eye sensitivity and yellowing of the irises, restlessness, tingling and incoordination.

The long-term impact upon my kidneys, liver, thyroid and other vital organs remains unknown, but perversely the most dangerous side effect related to the heart itself. As I understand it, beta-blocker and anti-arrhythmia medication stabilise its functioning by, amongst other things, reducing the flow of electrical activity triggering the ventricles to contract. In the first few weeks of experimentation during which dosage levels were optimised, there were occasions when my pulse and blood pressure fell so low that I was on standby for emergency treatment to stimulate the heart to beat faster – how ironic is that!

This illustrates one of the dilemmas of medical intervention which, at its worst, generates a vicious spiral of deterioration where presenting symptoms are treated with drugs or surgery which in turn generate side effects which then have to be treated causing further complications and so it goes on. This was the situation with my mother in the final stages of her struggle with cancer. She was undergoing a course of radiotherapy which, in addition to acting on the tumour, was damaging healthy tissue. Steroids were prescribed to counter these adverse effects which left her feeling nauseous, drastically depressing her appetite. As a consequence of not eating, she became too weak to continue with the radiotherapy with the inevitable consequences.

This is, perhaps, an extreme example, but there will be few of us who haven't experienced complications in one way or another – from a mild allergic reaction to a hospital-acquired infection. Most of them are minor and are readily offset by the benefits, but all remind us that medicine is not an exact science nor are its practitioners infallible. There is inherent risk involved in all treatment which can be minimised by diligent research and sound practice, but never eliminated. To deny as much is to delude ourselves and to place unreasonable expectations upon those who treat us. Although uncertainty is difficult to live with and raises the stakes considerably when it comes to placing our lives in the hands of doctors and the resources at their disposal, it is unavoidable and may even have a part to play in our healing by eliciting trust, thereby increasing receptivity to the creative possibilities residing beyond us in the skill of physicians, the therapeutic benefits of their treatments and the loving attention of those who care for us and will us to be well.

There is one final side effect which cannot go unmentioned. More often than not it's a consequence of being ill, although it can be triggered and certainly intensified by ensuing treatment. Depression is not so much a symptom as a condition in its own right, an instinctive and entirely understandable reaction to being wounded and crushed. Serious illness disrupts life. It stops us in our tracks, undermining our plans and aspirations, causing our worlds to shrink drastically and without warning. Suddenly, we are no longer able to do much of what previously filled our days, structuring our time whilst imbuing it with a sense of purpose and significance. Our circle of human interaction contracts. We become exiled from many of those whose colle-giality, friendship and presence enrich us. The satisfaction of a task accomplished, the edification of stimulating conversation, the affirmation of fulfilling a role, the anticipation of future prospects. All these are taken from us and we are left grieving their loss whilst pondering whether they will ever return or what will become of us if they don't.

It's difficult to express the sense of desolation that descended in the weeks following diagnosis as the impact of my condition began to impress itself. What is more, I feel awkward in mentioning it because, compared to the suffering of others, mine was superficial and inconsequential, yet depression is no respecter of such distinctions, falling indiscriminately upon the 'deserving' and 'innocent' alike. And once in place, it sucks all of life into its vortex of despond, blinding us to the good things that remain, clouding our judgement, weakening our will, eroding our confidence, starving us of hope – imposing upon us the victim's yoke. Languishing in an invisible prison, apathy soon sets in and with it despair over whether things will ever be other than they are, feeding an irrational suspicion of those 'light-bearers' who attempt to persuade us otherwise.

Yet, perhaps depression's deepest cut is its dishonesty. Like the anorexic who, looking in a mirror, is repulsed by the obese form that confronts, depression infects us with similar deceit. Two things saved me. A gratuitous tenacity refusing to be cast in depression's guise. And the faith, hope and love of others.

Chapter 9

Ministering Angels

I suppose it's just about possible to be ill in isolation, but for most of us it's a communal project. For one thing, unless content to lick our own wounds, we are drawn into a complex web of interactions with healthcare professionals and operatives. Each hospital is a microcosm of this phenomenon, staffed with a workforce of doctors, nurses, technicians, orderlies and administrators employed to attend to us. I think of it as a kind of theatre populated by actors improvising their roles according to a largely unwritten, though highly-regulated, script. Within the drama of our dis-ease, some have no more than walk-on parts whilst others are main stage, but even principal characters are substituted regularly. Inevitably, we relate to some of the cast better than others, although patient choice doesn't currently extend to selecting your troupe so it's best to be accommodating.

There is a hint of arranged marriages about this. We don't choose our medical attendees any more than they choose us. Instead, we're thrown together by circumstance and relate to one another through the parts we're given to play. So it matters little that we weren't acquainted beforehand. In fact, it probably helps. It establishes a certain detachment from the outset, reminding us that the kind of relating required of us is 'in role'. With time, of course, we become familiar, even friendly, and this can be a good thing, but I came to see it as a bonus rather than a right and one that shouldn't impinge upon our performance. After all, we expect professional service from staff members whether they like us or not; similarly, they expect us to cooperate and be civil in response.

This last point is worth amplifying. During a previous outing to A & E, this time in Sunderland, UK, I was surprised to find a metal grill on the reception counter as well as, throughout the waiting area, an ample supply of surveillance cameras, security guards and large signs specifying that abuse of staff, whether verbal or physical, wouldn't be tolerated. This puzzled me. After all, which of us would be so short-sighted as to harm those persons whose help we seek? I ended up spending the night in the A & E holding ward and was shocked by what transpired. One middle-aged man, admitted in an inebriated condition, treated the nurses appallingly – swearing, mocking, making sexual advances whilst demanding 'room service'. Then, after consuming a substantial breakfast, he discharged himself. A young woman arrived in the early hours accompanied by a 'minder' who, when a member of staff attempted to tidy their baggage into a locker, drew a knife and threatened to cut her up. The article in question contained illicit substances. The police were soon on the scene and arrests ensued. As they say, you couldn't make this stuff up. Within the space of a few hours, it became perfectly clear to me why it is that hospitals increasingly resemble prisons as I was left wondering whether a national health service is sustainable within a climate of exploitation and breakdown in trust – where those needing medical attention are unwilling or unable to embrace the responsibilities, as well as the privileges, of being a patient.

That New Year in Edinburgh, I found these constraints more of a help than a hindrance, supplying a code of conduct to moderate behaviour and inform interactions. Furthermore, the relative anonymity of relating 'in role' encourages candid exchange, with many of us finding it easier to be honest with a well-intentioned stranger than a family member or close friend. Somehow, it feels less complicated even though these encounters are often characterised by a level of intensity rarely matched elsewhere.

But there are potential pitfalls not least disparities over expectation and levels of personal investment. Let me explain by extending the theatrical analogy a little further. The measure of any actor is an ability to inhabit a role wholeheartedly and persuasively – to make it their own, drawing on professional training whilst offering a personal interpretation. When this happens, a performance possesses authority and verve; when absent, it becomes shallow and unconvincing. Although lacking relevant qualifications, patients probably have it easier in this respect for they are simply required to play themselves albeit within certain parameters. Medical staff, by contrast, have to adopt a persona which comes more naturally to some than to others, with predictable consequences. I am reminded of what the pig said to the hen as the farmer's wife prepared breakfast, "The difference between us is that whilst you have an interest in this operation, I'm fully committed!"

The first time I met our GP was on returning home from Edinburgh after being discharged from hospital. The health centre was new and buzzing, offering an impressive array of services. It had an air of friendly purposefulness about it – a 'lived-in' busyness where patients were related to as persons. Unlike those I had attended previously, you weren't summoned to a consulting room by a loudspeaker or electronic display; instead, doctors and nurses approached you in the waiting area. I was equally encouraged by the way my GP, having read through the discharge notes, set about investigating the symptoms for himself. Although this entailed further tests and procedures, including the now familiar bloodletting and ECG, it demonstrated a personal investment in my case as well as independence of mind.

Above all, though, I was reassured by his quality of attention. As a minister who was forever struggling to fit a quart into a pint pot, I learned the importance of giving yourself wholeheartedly to someone for the duration of each brief encounter. To put down the preoccupations of the past and the anticipations of the future in order to be present with that person and for that person. My doctor exhibited a similar commitment and one that extended beyond attending to a debilitating condition to supporting one of his patients through uncertain times and life-changing decisions. During the ensuing months, I frequently found myself in the doctor's surgery or the practice nurse's treatment room and on each occasion those first impressions were confirmed. Such visits will never rank among life's peak experiences. You wouldn't expect them to, but they were probably as good as it gets.

One thing about being overwhelmed is that you either sink without trace or find yourself buoyed up. It begins with drowning. In those early days of illness, it felt as if I was being sucked under by some leviathan bent on my destruction. Beginning to choke, well beyond the limits of my own resources, I realised to my amazement that I was still breathing. What made it all the more remarkable was that my oppressor hadn't been vanquished. Though still submerged within threatening circumstances, I was not starved of those life-giving substances capable of reviving the spirit and inspiring the soul. Nor was I truly 'at sea', at the mercy of the elements; somehow, I was being steered towards an undisclosed horizon where there would be shelter, sustenance and restoration – a destination yet to emerge from the chaos within and about.

My lifelines were multifarious. Emails, cards and letters, some brief, others discursive, expressing shock and concern, offering encouragement and support. Freshly cut flowers, dispersing colour and scent throughout ashen days, or a sumptuous sweetmeat to subdue the all-pervading taste of metal. Music, classical and contemporary, familiar and new, lightened the silence with texture and cadence. Stories, written or spoken, beckoned me to share in other lives and visit distant places. A miniature olive tree. All those gestures a failing memory reminds me I've forgotten. Each one particular yet all belonging to a common currency of grace embracing a gloriously catholic community of persons who, on learning of my misfortune, felt it had something to do with them. To be caught up within such a swell of compassion is surely among the most expansive of human experiences – the many expressions of goodwill possessing an enormity of their own, spilling into joyous incomprehension at the prospect of all those lives I had touched in some way.

To be the undeserving recipient of so much kindness is humbling. What is, perhaps, equally extraordinary is its capacity to sustain. Within this community, I was able to transcend the constraints of my predicament – to be myself within some former chapter characterised by a different set of circumstances. Their gifts acted as triggers, releasing memories flooding my consciousness. A CD of favourite tunes, a 'Fat Rascal' from *Betty's* cake shop, a parish magazine, postcards, photographs, reminiscences, local news, a cutting from the garden, something I had left behind, a task yet to be completed. Many of them bearing witness to the kind of instances we pass through without any inkling of their significance until someone bids us return, reminding us that we are each a part of one another's story.

Thankfully, wise guides were counted among them. Those who had weathered the storms, whose words carried particular authority. One letter comes to mind, typed and running to several pages. Its author also placed AF after her name. Like a seasoned pilot navigating treacherous seas, she described each symptom in such a way as to make it a place of meeting, revealing her own familiarity whilst confirming my own. Then, dispassionately and unpretentiously, she guided me through with practical advice, savvy counsel and purposeful intent. Not a whiff of pity, no window for self-indulgent sorrowing, without a hint of despondency. This was no communion of the hapless; rather, it was the summons of a teacher delivered with the gusto of a sergeant major: "Attention. You will survive. There is a way through. Trust me, I've been there." I've read Judith's letter a dozen times. Its confidence is infectious and guidance reassuring, but above all her testimony rescued me from self-doubt – I wasn't imagining it, the storm was real, but so was the lifeline.

There were phone calls, but relatively few and for understandable reasons. Inevitably, the immediacy of encounter is more exposing. Then there's the uncertainty over whether I would be up to fielding calls or, indeed, would welcome them. An implicit hierarchy comes into play determining the appropriate level of contact. I have sensed this myself in different circumstances – do I know this person sufficiently well to pick up the receiver and 'intrude'?

To begin with, phone calls were full of tears and silence. Somehow, uttering words and hearing voices without seeing faces concentrates emotions which, freed from the constraints of visibility and decorum, readily find expression through the inarticulate. Here, tears own a particular quality for, although unintentional (few of us choose to cry), they possess an honesty rarely equalled by the exchange of words. Such vulnerability is both an intimate confession and an invitation to similar intimacy. We have all known the awkwardness that tears can engender when that reciprocity cannot be responded to and they become a barrier to communication rather than a conduit. Yet when tears beget tears, when deep calls to deep, a meeting of souls ensues that is nothing short of sacramental.

Silence is rather more ambiguous. Sometimes it signals a loss of words where we are rendered speechless by what another person has said or by the circumstances surrounding respective lives. At other times, it discloses a measure of distraction accompanying those calls in which we haven't invested our full attention or where our focus is temporarily broken by some third party such as a doorbell, TV programme or new email (with that give-away ping!). But silence voluntarily inhabited is a fertile place where communion flourishes within the soils of impressionable sensitivity and attention.

With time, I became more attuned to the multidimensional texture of telephone communication and, somewhat impishly, devised a scheme of classification. For instance, there are *dutiful callers* who, spurred on by responsibility, commence with a purposeful "How are you?" in the hope of eliciting a similarly concise and upbeat reply – "I'm fine," "I'm on the mend," "Much improved, thank you." Less optimistic assessments or more detailed analysis tend to be greeted with incomprehension over how it could be taking so long, or galvanizing interjections such as "to hang on in there" or "to keep positive." The tempo tends to be brisk thereby reducing exposure to infection whilst catalysing rapid recovery. Silence, however brief, invariably signals the cessation of proceedings followed by sighs of relief all round – job done!

By contrast, *compassionate callers* are not seeking short-term returns and, as a consequence, are comfortable playing it long. The onset of tears is neither apologised for nor excused, but tacitly acknowledged as an integral part of communication. The tenor is that shared by travellers whose journeys converge for a season. Their companionship, understated yet sustaining, is characterised by lengthy tracts of silence punctuated by unhurried conversation which endures long after their paths separate.

Inquisitive callers are full of questions as they investigate the course of the illness to date as well as the nature and severity of current symptoms. Medication, consultations and treatment options are discussed at great length peppered with an ample supply of anecdotes and recommendations. A well-intentioned desire to understand sometimes verges on interrogation, as patients find themselves manufacturing details to satisfy inquiring minds, whilst the proffering of advice can come perilously close to coercion – "promise me you'll..." These calls rarely conclude naturally, but need to be ended by some form of interruption on the part of the recipient, who is left feeling exhausted, awkward and fearing offence may have been inadvertently caused.

Concerned callers seek reassurance. Their investment is intensely personal resulting in a pronounced sense of diminishment whenever a patient's illness is contemplated, sometimes to the point of fretfulness and depression. The world has become an unpredictable place as a dependable foundation within the caller's life has been destabilised. An unacknowledged exchange in roles often ensues in which patients become comforters and offer support to ameliorate the impact of their condition upon the affectionately-attached.

Then there are *preoccupied callers* who offer an initial greeting followed by an earnest inquiry into the patient's well-being before returning to familiar themes of their own circumstances. Competition for air space is almost always unsuccessful and runs contrary to the spirit of the exchange so the patient is best served by exercising patience through adopting the role of an active listener contributing the occasional prompt, expression of horror or affirming sound, as required.

No doubt, there are many other species within *genus telephonium* as well as mixed types. What a rich variety of communication the telephone is able to convey! This lighthearted and, yes, caricatured survey is not intended to be judgemental or dismissive, although I suspect we can all identify ourselves within it somewhere and some of us will be more comfortable with our pedigree than others. My point resides elsewhere, namely to recognise the small army of relations, friends, colleagues, parishioners, students and acquaintances who found a common cause in the desire to show solidarity and express concern – to offer me, and this applies equally to those who wrote or visited, the only commodity genuinely theirs to bestow – time. Whenever I reflect on this I feel a fresh surge of gratitude and appreciation that so many people were willing to interrupt their full and busy lives in this way.

Finally, let me say something about those whose presence was announced by the doorbell rather than a ringtone. Visits were relatively scarce during the first few weeks with many a prospecting phone call concluding a meeting to be premature. In most cases, this was a relief because I looked pretty awful, especially early on when the contrast between the 'then' and 'now' of my appearance was most pronounced. Those who did cross the threshold were invariably shocked by what they saw and struggled to disguise their feelings as their first reactions, raw, honest, uncut, made an impression no subsequent qualification could erase. I found the distress this caused painful and would do what I could to relieve any awkwardness. In many cases, it was the healing balm of laughter which proved to be a potent antidote and restorer of communion.

This was not the first time I had realised laughter's potential to liberate and subvert. I mentioned in an earlier chapter how I had nursed my mother during the final stages of cancer. This period spanned Christmas which raised the challenge of family celebrations. I recall agonizing over what would be an appropriate present. By then, she had been confined to bed for some time and was struggling with bedsores, cramps, muscle spasms and the like. What about an electric massager? It came to me as a eureka moment and, without further thought, one was acquired forthwith. On Christmas morning, the family gathered around Mother's bed to exchange gifts. With a little assistance, she managed to unwrap my offering and to switch it on. Not only did it resemble something from an Ann Summers' catalogue, but when she applied it to an aching region of her anatomy, cancer had so ravaged her body that it reverberated against her bones like a stick striking a taut drum skin. It was tragic to witness as the severity of her condition struck us with renewed force; but this death sentence was eclipsed by the absurdity of supplying Mother with a vibrating dildo-lookalike for Christmas. We were all reduced to tears, they were tears of laughter – transfiguring the awesome prospect of parting, allowing a little light, warmth and hopefulness to flood in.

I also struggled with the well-intentioned 'cotton wool' and 'kid gloves' approach that often accompanied first visits and would endeavour to reassure cautious callers that my ticker was unlikely to stop in the near future nor would I shatter into a million pieces if dropped on the floor. To allay fears further I would withdraw into the kitchen only to re-emerge forthwith carrying (somewhat unsteadily) a small tray of refreshments. This tended to do the trick, especially if there was chocolate cake to distract attention on to matters gastronomic.

It's fascinating, though, to reflect on how we respond to those we know when they've been transformed into patients. More often than not our overriding aim is to express concern, offer support and show sensitivity so we don't inadvertently make things worse. But it's far from easy to accomplish. For one thing, what patients long for from their visitors more than anything else is normality – to be related to as persons not cases. A visit is a rare opportunity to break curfew – to breathe fresh air in the company of ordinary people who have come to share their days or muse about what has been happening elsewhere.

For this reason, more edifying liaisons tended to be those where conversation extended beyond symptoms, side effects and hospital interiors to focus on something refreshingly non-medical for which the adoption of hushed tones or a sanitised poise was unnecessary – where talk was spontaneous, expansive and preoccupying. Sometimes, meetings with work colleagues developed in this fashion – business to attend to, recommendations to make, decisions to reach. Friends relating holiday reminiscences also proved fruitful in this respect so long as it didn't involve viewing video footage which, in my experience, tends to be barely more engaging than watching reality TV. By contrast, listening to animated voices recounting exploits and impressions can be fascinating.

For the most part, I was content to listen. Talking precipitated fatigue, but more importantly I was bored with my predicament and had no desire to bore others with it. Visits were too important for that. They afforded an all too infrequent opportunity to enjoy company once more and, through doing so, to inhabit the fuller self that illness threatened to destroy. More so, I came to see listening as a gift of attention, even though I wasn't very adept and often dozed off – something of worth to offer my guests along with decaffeinated tea and goodies from the Tupperware container. It mattered that those who came would not look upon it as a waste of time. I could not expect my visitors to enjoy themselves, but hoped that our encounters were not beyond mutual enrichment.

This has been the longest chapter to date and intentionally so. I wanted to underline the importance of other people and to illustrate some of the ways in which they've contributed to the healing process – from medical professionals employed for this purpose to passing acquaintances who, on learning of my situation, felt moved to respond. Interestingly, one of the words used in the Bible for 'compassion' literally means 'to be moved in the bowels'. Lest this be misunderstood, we need to recall how the bowels used to be considered the seat of the emotions and for good reason – without becoming overly anatomical, there is something about the powerful stirrings of this region that captures compassion's claim over us.

One final thing, as a clergyman, you would expect like-minded supporters "to say one for me." And so they did. What I found remarkable, though, was just how many people from every point on the compass of religious belief volunteered their prayers. This set me thinking – was this a parcel of 'goodwill' wrapped in language I would find familiar and comforting or was there more to it? I've long maintained that praying is instinctive. In certain contexts, often when confronting circumstances beyond our control or comprehension, we find it going on within us. It may well not be a conscious choice, but it's happening nonetheless almost as if the propensity to pray is hard-wired into our humanity. Perhaps it is. Perhaps we no more invented praying than we did breathing. In truth, our inventiveness depends upon both. But to whom or what are we praying and what do we hope our prayers will accomplish? These are important although, I've come to believe, secondary concerns for which there are as many answers as there are prayers. What matters is that we're praying or, rather, that there's praying going on within us.

I appreciate little about how my breathing keeps me alive beyond the fact that it does. Prayer is not so different. Like every breath we inhale, it bears witness to our humility, which is another word with an insightful derivation, coming from the Latin root *humus* meaning 'soil' or 'earth', as does the word humanity. Praying, like breathing, reminds us that we are children of clay, dependent and contingent beings. Whatever else illness achieves, it restores perspective by demonstrating beyond contradiction that, for all our protestations to the contrary, we are not controllers of our destiny, but vulnerable creatures at the mercy of the exigencies of time and presences beyond our invention, yet inherently susceptible to grace.

Chapter 10

Companions

One person conspicuous by her absence from the previous chapter is my wife, Liz. This was no oversight, but in recognition that the impact of my illness upon her life has been qualitatively different to those mentioned so far. Had we been able to start a family, our children would belong here as well. As it is, I will say something later about the other living being sharing our space, namely Tess, our golden retriever.

"For better, for worse, for richer, for poorer, in sickness and in health, to love and to cherish, till death us do part ..." when Liz and I made our marriage vows back in 1982, we had every intention of keeping them but little idea what that would entail. No one entering into a lifelong relationship does. However strong the emotional attraction and the confidence it engenders, it is always a leap of faith, a risky one at that, grounded in love's capacity to sustain covenant. To a measure, this is what distinguishes how partners experience the illness of their 'other halves'. They don't choose to express concern and offer support in the same way as those ministering angels celebrated in the previous chapter; rather, our partners suffer it personally not by contracting it (although this sometimes happens), but because their lives, inextricably linked with ours, become implicated by it.

Although it's for Liz to relate her half of the story, let me reflect a little on how she has appeared throughout this ordeal. Perhaps the place to start is with her encouragement to seek medical help in the first instance. If you remember, it was her gentle prompting which resulted in that providential phone call to *NHS 24*. This has been characteristic of her companionship – attention, encouragement and challenge. She noticed something was up and enabled me to reach the same conclusion. This may seem unremarkable, but when both of you are immersed in demanding careers, spending little time together, it was perceptive and apposite – permission to take myself seriously in the midst of all the claims upon my waking hours.

Whether Liz was consciously aware of doing this I rather doubt; it was yet another expression of love's evolving vernacular animating the covenant between us. Much of her response belongs here within the sphere of what may be described as instinctive intention. This sounds like a contradiction in terms, but it isn't. Think of parents who, on hearing their children's cries, drop what they are doing and make haste to assist. Or of a footballer who, without looking up, threads the ball through to his unmarked teammate. In neither case is a decision knowingly made, but both are expressions of a skilled intuitive relationship, rooted in commitment – informing perception, shaping behaviour.

As I say, this is where I locate much of Liz's response. It was characteristic of her way of being and relating more generally. In this respect, my illness was no less revealing for her than for me. On the whole, I found this reassuring because it reflected her stability in crisis as well as her unflappable temperament. I didn't expect Liz to be overawed by what happened or to wrap me in tissue paper or to gaze despairingly into an uncertain future. That isn't her way. Instead, she applied herself with purposefulness and resolve, acknowledging the seriousness of the situation whilst refusing to be governed by it, showing solidarity without becoming sentimental or pitying and, above all, maintaining access to those surpluses of existence, the extraordinary ordinariness of love's routines and vernacular, which characterised our life together and transcended present constraints.

One unexpected blessing in this last respect was the opportunity to spend more time together. Up to this point, home life had been more an appealing prospect than a lived-in reality. For much of our marriage, Liz has spent up to four nights per week away with work and, when she was in residence, we regularly remained 'in harness' from eight in the morning until around ten o'clock at night when we aimed to share our main meal of the day together in the kitchen with the *Ten O'Clock News* team. Things were a little less rigorous at the weekend, but not much. That is one of the implications of being a member of the clergy. Sundays are working days, rarely with less than three services and sometimes with as many as seven, whilst Saturdays tended to fill up with weddings, sermon preparation and various church-based events. So much for vicars only working one day a week. I wish!

All this changed in January. Whilst attempting some job-related task most days, whatever mental energy I could muster was spent long before Liz returned home sometime after seven. My inability to work into the evening encouraged her to close down by eight-thirty when we would supper together in the lounge (a room rarely visited beforehand) in front of the screen. When your staple diet consists of chicken salad, *MasterChef* was an instant success with each mouthful of lettuce transformed into some culinary delight appearing before our eyes. With one or two exceptions, though, we rapidly gave up on the TV listings shifting our allegiance to DVD sets. More entertaining evenings than I can remember were spent in the company of President Bartlet and the staff of the White House as we worked our way through seven seasons of *The West Wing*. Then we discovered *24*, the high-octane exploits of federal agent Jack Bauer and the Los Angeles Counter-Terrorist Unit. This was edge-of-the-seat stuff with many a forkful of food ending up in free fall as unexpected developments had us jumping out of our skins.

We soon began to look forward to these times which, in turn, developed their own rituals. One that will horrify conscientious dog-owners relates to dessert when Tess would join us on the couch for a plate of fresh fruit (previously sliced) before taking her post-prandial nap on Liz's lap. There was nothing remarkable about these evenings, but they became little oases of domesticity when we could recreate together. As the months passed, their therapeutic value also emerged as the stresses and strains of our situation dissipated amidst the crunching of apples and the affairs of state unfolding on the other side of the Pond.

For all this, it was Liz's ability to maintain normality that proved invaluable. I've already commented on how illness not only debilitates, but also threatens to infect all aspects of a sufferer's life as well as those who share in it. I was determined from the outset to prevent this from happening. From the first night in hospital when Liz was persuaded to return to base rather than mount a bedside vigil, I have encouraged her to continue with 'business as usual' wherever possible. Of course, there were numerous occasions when I missed her reassuring presence and others when I yearned to be able to get on with my life as she was getting on with hers. But for the most part I drew strength from the knowledge that her routines and work commitments remained largely unaffected. Her departure each morning and homecoming each night provided a framework for my days as much as for hers. And when she returned there would be another of those expansive rituals of ordinariness: catching up on each other's days, with news from beyond the limits of my world supplying at least one party with an edifying tonic. Financially, we would have struggled to make ends meets without Liz's employment and been forced to implement major lifestyle adjustments, including moving house amidst the throes of a housing recession, which would have brought more trauma and disruption. Above all, by maintaining a measure of independence, Liz bore witness to our life unaffected by illness. She remained free to be and her freedom loosened my shackles too.

Which brings me to Tess. I've often wondered whether the claim that dogs resemble their owners holds true in our case.

Certainly, there are similarities, notably when it comes to enthusiasm, freedom of spirit and love of food, but in other areas it's not so obvious. For example, Tess has more hair in one square inch of her coat than I boast on my entire head, whilst I hope a propensity for sniffing lampposts and the posteriors of fellow canines wasn't inherited from me. Be that as it may, one area where she felt the impact of my illness was walkies. Around Christmas, Tess' exercise regime dropped from two hearty outings per day to a couple of brief meanderings up the lane to attend to calls of nature. Where once our pace made little provision for wayside snuffling now there was ample time as she waited for me to catch up. And her girth soon revealed as much for whilst the burning of calories had drastically reduced the same could not be said for her appetite.

What I find significant here is that even at my lowest ebb, breathless and struggling with chronic fatigue, we went out. Irrespective of the weather, however brief and unsatisfactory, daily outings were non-negotiable. When illness had denuded my diary of almost everything, one of the few mainstays was the collar and the lead. I remember a sense of inner resolve to persevere with this 'rebellion' come what may. For some reason never articulated this was to be my line in the sand. In retrospect, it isn't so difficult to see why. Outings with Tess were habitual and brought to each day expectation and routine. Necessary also in as much as I owed Tess a duty of care which, in turn, provided a source of motivation. Walks could be measured and timed enabling me to plot progress or the lack of it. But, above all, they represented the exercising of choice – within all the constraints of my situation this was something I chose to do. How vital this is – whether sick or healthy, captive or free – that there is a door for which we alone possess the key and determine whether it stands locked or open.

Tess supplied much more than an excuse for donning my walking shoes. She was another companion – a creaturely presence who shared the journey and, sometimes, the struggle. We took it in turns to set the route, although Tess was much better at anticipating mine than vice versa. Apart from one or two tricky bits where the lead was necessary, we travelled unattached, lost in our own preoccupations. Then, every so often, we would converge for a stroke or the odd biscuit or to delight in the wind filling our faces or the scenery filling our eyes. Once we were meandering down a nearby lane when a huge rabbit leapt on to a drystone wall no more than feet away. Tess and I were rapt with wonder and surprise. I cannot imagine what those excursions would have been like without her; in truth, they wouldn't have taken place. For without the unspoken communion of companions filling the interstices between steps, walking can compound our loneliness. And journeys shared tend to traverse different terrain and reach different destinations to those undertaken alone.

Another source of company, more subtle, took the form of audiobooks. Having trudged through a few mountainous tomes on history and philosophy, I roamed into the fertile foothills of novels and biographies. These other lives transported me to unfamiliar cultures set in places previously no more than names on a map where I travelled along the traces left by other people's footprints – seeing, hearing, experiencing, occupying their place and time – realising I could still feel, that compassion hadn't deserted me.

One book proved to be particularly rewarding, *A Thousand Splendid Suns*, by Khaled Hosseini. Set in Afghanistan during the second half of the twentieth century, it relates the harrowing story of Mariam as she struggles to eke out an existence amidst austere conditions and an oppressive Taliban regime whilst yoked to a brutal husband, who abuses her in every way. However, one of Rasheed's attempts at humiliation, taking another wife, eventually backfires when Mariam and Laila become the closest of friends, sharing the love between a mother and a daughter. At last, Mariam has discovered something, someone, worth living for. Through their relationship, a measure of healing and restoration takes place as she recovers a sense of self-worth which, in turn, empowers her to break free from her oppressors and to sacrifice her life for the sake of her beloved.

The quality of characterisation, description and storyline create a narrative world in which I found myself participating not simply as an interested bystander, but as someone whose life had become entwined with the lives being played out within these pages. Like a vivid dream, I belonged to their story. Listening on my MP3 player (the novel is beautifully narrated by Atossa Leoni), there were occasions when I was overwhelmed by what transpired, engendering tears, empathy and sorrow, disbelief, indignation and revulsion, insight, appreciation and introspection, foreboding, fear and relief, smells, tastes and touches, voices, images and impressions. I emerged a different person through my encounter with Mariam, Laila, Jalil and Rasheed. It had been anything but an easy listen; somehow, though, I managed to stay the distance and sense I am a richer person for having done so – my humanity expanded in that way profound experience affords.

Good literature possesses that enlightening, transformative capacity. Each narrative relating a journey on which we are accompanied by the *dramatis personae* populating the plot. They too become our companions as we are thrown together by circumstance. To begin with there is strangeness. The book alone supplies the grounds for our acquaintance. Yet, as we proceed through the pages, a kind of relating takes place. Personalities come into focus. We share in the unfolding of their stories, step by step. Their passions and preoccupations, exploits and routines, preferences and prejudices, intimate thoughts and unfettered ambitions, relationships and liaisons, become ours. Whether they attract or intrigue us, baffle or beguile us, infuriate or repulse us, when the final full stop signals the parting of our ways few of us are the same persons as when we commenced.

No value can be placed on what has been spoken of in this and the previous chapter. The 'others' who rescued me not so much from a failing heart, which is no more than a biological malfunction, but from the ensuing personal diminishment and isolation. Where would we be without companions? In truth, who would we be? But there is one more of whom I must attempt to speak.

Chapter 11

Befriending the 'Enemy'

Once the initial diagnosis had been made back in January the game plan was clear. Medicate to reduce the pulse rate, stabilise the heart and thin the blood. Then, with the risk of clots forming reduced, restore the heart's normal rhythm using drugs or more invasive procedures – containment then cure. It would take weeks rather than days, but at least there was a strategy for returning me to work within a manageable time frame. In terms of my employment, it was inconvenient, especially as I had only recently taken up a new appointment, but manageable thanks to supportive colleagues and understanding students. Before then, there was little likelihood of improvement because everything, it appeared, depended on my heart operating satisfactorily. Meanwhile, it was a matter of learning to live within constraints.

This proved to be easier said than done, not least because I would only resign myself to the realities of the situation once I had struggled to accomplish as much as I could in terms of my job and those subsistence tasks of everyday existence. This resulted in a daily pattern in which, having returned from whatever I could manage by way of a walk with Tess, I would plug away at my desk until falling asleep or becoming so exasperated by my lack of progress that I gave up. Then followed sizeable periods spent in a twilight zone between consciousness and unconsciousness where I was unable to focus on anything for more than a few minutes at a time and then only superficially. Respite took the form of human interaction including regular visits to the health centre or hospital.

What made this period all the more unsatisfactory was its open-endedness. The rate-determining factor was anticoagulation. No attempt to restore the heart's normal rhythm could be contemplated until the viscosity of my blood had been reduced. Without becoming over-technical, this is measured by a convention known as the International Normalized Ratio (INR) and monitored by regular blood samples. I had been given a target INR of 2.5, but for some reason my system proved particularly resistant to the effects of warfarin used to achieve this goal. This resulted in a number of weeks when dosage was increased substantially with little or no effect. I ended up on levels that would have dangerously inflated most people's INR scores. What is more, it had taken over two months to achieve what for many patients can be accomplished in a matter of days. Finally, by the beginning of March, the elusive INR of 2.5 was reached and we were able to move beyond damage limitation to restorative treatment. It sounds like a major achievement; it was nothing of the sort.

The Consultant prescribed a potent anti-arrhythmia drug in the first instance. This would stabilise the heart and in some cases caused it to revert to normal operation without further action. Needless to say, this didn't happen in my case so we resorted to Plan B, electro cardioversion, where the heart is shocked back into sinus rhythm by applying an electrical charge with the aid of defibrillators. Like most medical procedures, it doesn't pay to ponder too closely what actually happens, although resuscitation scenes from screenplays kept springing to mind. Instead, I sought solace in the knowledge that it would be executed under general anaesthetic – at least I would be oblivious to it all!

The cardioversion was scheduled for the following week. I turned up in the morning, donned the requisite back-fastening surgical gown and wended my way to the operating theatre where I was introduced to the cast before taking up position on the table. The anaesthetist applied the knockout drops before asking me how I felt. "Fiiiiiiiine," I replied. The next thing I remember was being back in the ward with a couple of scald marks on my chest. I didn't bother inquiring where they had come from – my imagination supplied the answer. All I needed to know was that the procedure had been successful. The atrial flutter had flown. Normal transmission had been resumed.

Naively, I expected to feel better almost immediately. This untimely episode had already consumed a large enough bite out of my life. Naturally, it would take a little while for the anaesthetic to wear off and for my body to recover from being connected to the mains. But surely, I thought, this would be a matter of days. After all, if the heart is a pump and mine had not been working properly, now that it was, improvement would rapidly ensue. Then there were those testimonies of fellow-sufferers which spoke of overnight transformations and new leases of life. It was hardly surprising, then, that my expectations were high which made what followed even more disappointing.

It was not all bad news. After three or four weeks, my physical strength started to pick up. Tess and I were trotting once more and the duration of our outings increased from a few minutes to the best part of an hour. However, this was the exception rather than the rule. Other debilitating symptoms persisted. Mental fatigue, poor concentration and memory difficulties, together with other impaired cognitive functioning, proved particularly resilient, rendering reading and writing all but impossible. Conversation and human interaction of any kind left me drained, whilst nausea and headaches caused me to wake early each morning before accompanying me through the day. I will refrain from mentioning the raft of little handicaps that cumulatively made the performance of straightforward tasks a struggle.

But what was the cause? To start with, my blood pressure and pulse were abnormally low. There were abnormalities in my blood also. Then there was the possibility of side effects from medication. Further tests ensued. We decided to risk a phased withdrawal of the drugs and, whilst my heart remained in rhythm, there was little sign of progress. Through it all, I was aware of my status changing once more as the patient's dignity bestowed by diagnosis, justifying one's condition, was swept from under my feet, reducing me to a nomad wandering through a desert of unexplained symptoms. This affected me deeply. I found myself sinking into a mire of introspection and self-doubt. Was I imaging things? Should I call on the services of a psychiatrist? Or would a firm kick to my posterior do the trick? It was a harrowing time when seemingly every attempt to escape my predicament resulted in abject failure. And as the siege continued, it became increasingly apparent that I couldn't hold out much longer on making a decision about my employment. Then that moment arrived.

You may recall me mentioning that I had recently started a new job. After twelve full and fruitful years serving as a parish priest in the north-east of England, the previous autumn I had taken over responsibility for a training course in West Yorkshire tasked with preparing adults for ordained ministry, principally within the Church of England – a 'vicar factory' as one teenager from my former watch described it. Like most new appointments, my first term entailed a steep learning curve as I adapted to a different culture, work pattern and set of expectations. It had been an exhilarating and productive few months yielding a good deal of positive feedback. All of which confirmed our decision to leave Tyneside when we did. Then, before the year was out, a promising start was frustrated by illness. No sooner had I begun to establish myself in a new role than I was forced to withdraw. It felt so unfair, so futile, compelling me to let our students down whilst placing extra burdens on my colleagues. What made it even more problematic was that the course was in the midst of significant change and needed someone to keep a guiding hand on the tiller. That person was supposed to be me.

I cannot tell you how frustrating and demoralizing this proved to be. It felt as if some alien vessel had launched a torpedo in our direction when we had only just embarked on a new voyage, leaving us reeling. My relatively brief period in post coupled with the transitional phase in the course's evolution meant I couldn't afford to be off sick for more than a few weeks. I suspect the powers-that-be realised as much even though most parties opted to pretend otherwise or at least to keep their own counsel. However, when the weeks became months and a firm diagnosis with a predictable outcome gave way to a tranche of debilitating symptoms whose cause remained elusive and duration impossible to determine, the writing was on the wall. In my own mind, I had worked out a date by which there needed to be sufficient signs of improvement to give confidence that, at the very latest, I would be fit and ready to reengage by the beginning of the new academic year. The calculation was based on how long it would take to appoint a replacement and, hence, when the process needed to be underway.

That date duly came around, regrettably unaccompanied by those eagerly anticipated signs of recovery. In consequence, it no longer seemed responsible to prolong my absence further. A meeting with the chair of the Governing Body was hastily convened at which I tendered my resignation on the grounds of ill health. Reluctantly, it was accepted. After struggling to stay afloat, the ship had finally gone under and, with it, my hopes and aspirations.

Whatever energy I could muster during the ensuing weeks was devoted to managing the repercussions. The expressions of surprise, solidarity and sadness were reassuring and disheartening in equal measure. It was encouraging to discover I had made a positive impression, but this only deepened the sense of loss and regret. Perversely, the process of disengagement proved to be distracting in a positive way in that it enabled me to focus on other people once more. However, this inevitably dissipated as the reality of my predicament reasserted itself, only this time it seemed more daunting than ever in the absence of a firm diagnosis or the security of a job.

I had become a misplaced person whom the medical profession was unable to accommodate yet who remained unable to return 'home' to work. My GP began to suspect chronic fatigue syndrome. I wondered whether recovery would ever come or whether this was as good as it was going to get. It surprised me how my capacity to manage a set of symptoms depended on the framework in which they were set. Whilst they belonged to a diagnosis of a curable condition, I endured them as temporary inconveniences and did whatever I could to precipitate their departure. Now they threatened to settle in for good.

This threw me into a quandary. Was I someone who was recovering or who had recovered? Was I in the process of being restored to health or had that process run its course? At first, answering these questions seemed essential and determinative, affecting my status as a person. With time, though, these options began to look less defined as it dawned on me that health is always relative, with no absolute benchmarks. None of us is completely well (in truth, I am not sure what that would mean) for we are constantly exposed to the processes of decay that surround us and are embedded within our genetic make-up. We strive to keep them at bay and may recover to a measure from skirmishes incurred along the way, but in the end they prevail. For each of us inhabits a continuum stretching from the vitality associated with birth to the inertia characterising death. At any one instant we rest somewhere within these limits. Age is but one factor as those sprightly octogenarians who jog by confirm; and some of us are closer to death when in the prime of life. What is more, because we're complex, multidimensional creatures, different 'parts' of us will be more energised or dis-eased than others. As I say, it's relative.

Such considerations didn't entirely reconcile me to my situation nor take away the longing to feel better than I did, but they aided in a process of accepting there was no going back. No return to pre-12/31. No period of convalescence, however long or productive, would be able to undo what had taken place because every assault mounted by the forces of decay scars us, weakens us, changes us – yet, paradoxically, possesses the capacity to enrich us as well. Being healthy for me could no longer mean striving to be 'now' what I was 'then'. Life had moved on. I had moved on. The events of the past months belonged to me. The challenge was no longer whether they could be eradicated (patently, they couldn't), but whether they could be incorporated into my human being.

It is no coincidence that 'integrate' and 'integrity' share the same Latin root, meaning 'sound, whole, complete', suggesting that our integrity (or wholeness) resides in being able to integrate all the fragments of living composing the biography that is you or me. To hold them together in creative tension, like voices in a debating chamber or instruments in a jazz ensemble, so that the glory of the whole emerges from the investment of the parts. But more so, and here a further metaphor is needed, to allow the various ingredients of our lives to blend together, illness included. And, through doing so, to discover that even the most unpalatable ones when experienced 'neat' can, like salt, season the entire dish. Increasingly, I've come to see this integrating process as vital to our healing and wholeness.

Befriending the 'enemy'. I am aware this sounds counter-intuitive, even outrageous. After all, illness tends to come upon us in an untimely manner and against our wills. It invades our space and hijacks our lives, holding us hostage. The ensuing suffering can be alien, pernicious, threatening. We feel dis-eased and diminished. How can this possibly be wholesome or good?

Instinctively, I relate to this response, but find the image of wholeness to which it bears witness unsatisfactory, namely that health is principally about inoculation, isolation and purification – about absence rather than presence. It's about *not* becoming ill, separating ourselves from potential sources of contagion and purging the body whenever it becomes infected. This seems a rather impoverished view and one which discloses more about what we are trying to avoid than what we seek to embrace or, indeed, to become. It is symptomatic, I think, of what can be described as the *lifeboat approach* to living where we strive to pass through the waters of existence protected from the elements and safe from danger. To further this goal, we populate our lives with low-risk, like-minded individuals whilst avoiding as many hazards as possible. If all goes to plan, we are duly rewarded with an easy passage and longevity to boot.

But isn't health more than this, more than absence? The recent ascendancy of terms such as 'well-being' or 'wellness' suggests as much. Often, though, they are equated with little more than feelings or states of mind. For instance, the leisure industry promotes a positive image of health in terms of feeling good about yourself and positive about your prospects. It's about looking after Number One and maximizing your potential. "What's wrong with that?" I hear you say. Only that it assumes the pursuit of health is essentially an individualistic vocation – something we achieve by ourselves, for ourselves. Other people are involved, of course, but only in as much as they are useful *to us*, serving as 'means' to our 'ends'.

To my mind, this doesn't ring true. I long to be healthy as much as the next person, but am convinced that it cannot be achieved in isolation. We need others, not principally to make us feel good, further our life goals or protect us from harm, but to expand our humanity by drawing us into relationships of mutuality and respect. Relationships where our sense of personal identity and worth (as well as theirs) are informed by those whose lives touch ours – who belong, as we do, to a web of inter-connectedness and reciprocity. Relationships that only become possible when we abandon the lifeboat and dare to swim in the sea of our common humanity where we are exposed to the harsh realities of existence and the vagaries of experience, as well as to the fathomless capacities of personal encounter.

Here, it seems to me, is a vision of health which resonates with our deepest core. For we are relationally-constituted beings. We need others to be fully, authentically ourselves. In truth, there is a part of each of us residing in another's gift which only emerges as we risk ourselves to encounter. From this perspective, health is about wholeness and integrity, about integration within and without. And the pursuit of this takes us beyond cures to life's ills or protection from them in the first place to passionate engagement in a world full of surprises – some good, some ill – where we discover that we are related to people we had never heard of and situations or issues we once blocked from our minds.

Whatever else may emerge from my experience of being a patient, I've gained a fuller appreciation of the nature of wholeness – integration and encounter: gathering together the fragments of our lives, openness to others. Central to both is being related, that is human being formed from the tapestry of life's experiences and those persons who belong to them. Jim Cotter, a seasoned pioneer in this field, puts it like this:

The whole of me, the whole person, physical, mental, emotional, spiritual, is in need of being healed, of being made whole. The curing of physical symptoms is but one part of this process: the absence of cure need not hinder it. My own healing is bound up with that of others. I need to pray and work for the healing of the nations, for food for the hungry, for justice for the downtrodden, for my neighbours in a global village. Without their well-being I cannot be completely well.
– *Healing – More or Less* (Sheffield: Cairns, 1990), pp. 1–5

Chapter 12

Entrusting

When I started to record these reflections, it was my intention to keep going until fully recovered. Much has happened since then not least in relation to my perception of being a patient. Along the way, I've discovered healing is not the same as being cured, and wholeness is a way of being that is accessible to us in times of illness as much as when we're feeling fine and dandy. In truth, it constitutes the integrity that is our inheritance and vocation.

This needs a little unpacking. Let me begin with a word about what I am not affirming. This isn't a remix of the *Patience Strong* theme where a stiff upper lip is prescribed for all of life's misfortunes. There's something archetypically English about this outlook encapsulated in those war movies where the officer emerges from the fray carrying a wounded comrade whilst some part of his own anatomy is hanging off who, when medical assistance is offered, replies "It's nothing, really." What I find unsatisfactory about this approach is that it takes neither the sufferer nor the suffering seriously. The truth is bad things do happen and they hurt. We are not immunised against their poison by refusing to acknowledge their existence or struggling on regardless. The woman who feels a lump in her breast and does nothing about it. The husband who refuses to accept his wife is dead. Children who remain silent about their abuse. The person with flu who goes to work or school anyway. There may be extenuating circumstances for such courses of action, but eventually the malady festers or spreads until its presence can no longer be ignored.

Nor am I advocating a *batten down the hatches* approach where we take to the lifeboats as per the previous chapter or cultivate a kind of detachment through becoming desensitized to what happens to us or to those around us. I recognise this can be the only short-term strategy for survival when confronting some of life's inhumanities. But it is inherently diminishing because through cutting ourselves off from sources of hurt we are in danger of cutting ourselves off from potential sources of healing also. For instance, victims of torture, betrayal or, for that matter, infectious diseases may, quite understandably, seek refuge within an inner sanctum beyond the reach of aggressive intruders. Yet, by doing so, they risk unintentionally compounding their suffering by sentencing themselves to self-imposed solitary confinement.

No, what I've come to realise is that being a patient simply accentuates the nature of being human, namely that we are vulnerable creatures for whom suffering is an inevitable conse-quence of our frailty. For all our protestations, we can no more escape it than we can make ourselves immortal. In this respect, death is the great reality-test, finalising a process that commenced the moment our body clocks started ticking. As Bob Dylan memorably penned, "he not busy being born is busy dying" (*It's Alright, Ma*). This is not as depressing as it sounds – for if it is true then it belongs to us, is a part of our story. Death clarifies the nature of our existence, frames it and thereby concentrates our experience of living. Or, at least, has the potential to do so.

But there is more, for the reason why we suffer and die is also the means by which we can find healing, wholeness, peace. If we are susceptible to those corrosive forces from without then equally we are able to enter into covenant with those life-giving presences beyond our making. We are, after all, relationally-constituted beings who find our integrity within a web of inter-connectedness and reciprocity. We need others to be ourselves. This was the saving grace of my illness. Those conduits of love, care and concern that sustained through suffering, reassuring me that there was more to my life than atrial flutter and a basketful of debilitating symptoms defying diagnosis – that within this failing frame resided something, someone of worth – a person who mattered, who was a part of and belonged to other persons and their stories. This reality didn't suddenly come into existence that New Year's Eve. My incapacity simply enabled those lifelines submerged within the busyness of our days to surface and take the strain. But once they did, their presence proved robust and enduring, supplying energising resources every bit as essential in their own way as those passing through an umbilical cord in a mother's womb.

And through all this I have been aware of another covenant. There was nothing so tangible as a card or visit; its presence was subtle and ambiguous. I couldn't point to any one thing and say, "That's what I'm talking about," and yet it infused much of what mattered as the air we breathe carries the voices of our conversations: in the back of the ambulance en route to A & E... during moments of acute loneliness and depression... resonating through expressions of loving concern or hope-filled good wishes... underpinning the physician's art, the onset of spring, the rhythm of each day or a beating heart... inspiring the swallow's dance, the taste of freshly picked raspberries, the abandonment of laughter and every surplus of our existence... inhabiting the confusion, the frustration, the silence, the suffering.

It was a kind of companionship, a subtle communing personal in nature, with one who was wholly other yet wholly present – a presence amplified by those persons, events and experiences I've just alluded to and yet transcending them. Is this wishful thinking? Perhaps, but probably not. For the same reason that there is all the difference in the world between being in love with being in love and being in love with someone who is in love with you. At times, they may appear identical but the former will never surprise us nor draw us into a fuller sense of self. Through all the diminishment of the past months, I've emerged with a deeper appreciation of the extraordinary gratuitousness of life, together with an uncanny conviction that the truth about my own existence resides in this mysterious otherness who is beyond us, within us and around us.

Of course, I cannot prove this nor should I wish to try. It would, in any case, be a futile pursuit bearing the seeds of its own destruction through excluding the one means by which we are able to stumble into God. Forgive another 'partner' analogy. Would I be more inclined to trust Liz if I employed the services of a private investigator to track her every move when out of sight? I suspect not because the desire to demonstrate her trustworthiness would, in effect, be evidence of my unwillingness or, at least, inability to trust her in the first place. There is, in my experience, no way to circumvent trust's inherent riskiness nor the vulnerability to which it exposes us. Yet, whilst those whom we trust cannot be scrutinised as objects, our trust can be confirmed retrospectively as we inhabit its communion and grow into those expanses of human being to which it gives access.

This is why I discern something more in all that I have related in these pages – expressions of an enduring love animated and embodied in the countless acts of kindness, generosity and goodwill extended to me. Daily entrusting my life to the source of this enduring love, to the ground of our being, whilst perceiving its presence in those around me, has been integral to my healing. What is more, these months of illness have engendered within me that most fundamental and fruitful of human orientations by which we are able to encounter not only one another but also the one whom we call God – trust.

In drawing the threads together in this way, I claim no privilege. In fact, although a priest for over twenty years, public worship, formal prayer and bible reading, with a few notable exceptions, have been conspicuous by their absence during my illness. However, I haven't been without a guide. It was back in my early twenties, as related earlier, whilst reading the works of the great existential thinkers that the harsh realities of life – those truths we would rather ignore about death and decay, human frailty and depravity, life's inherent meaninglessness and futility – impressed themselves with devastating clarity and force. Buckling under their enormity, I became profoundly aware of something more, a reality capable of embracing even the pathetic tragedy of the human predicament.

I had been a professing Christian for many years by then, but it had been a matter of belief – believing certain things about God, Christ, sin, the Bible, the sacraments, heaven and hell, salvation and the rest. But when staring death in the face, these beliefs – as substantial and well founded as they once appeared – seemed to evaporate before my eyes, leaving me naked and exposed, yet extraordinarily open and receptive. It was then that I first recognised there is only one response that defines us absolutely as human beings. Trust – simple, uncompromising, all-embracing – which finds its ultimate expression in a readiness to risk all that we are to all who God is – to place our lives in God's hands – without knowing whether such a God exists beyond the limits of our imaginations.

In the ambulance last New Year's Eve, it defined my existence once more. Only this time it was more familiar because of a deepening acquaintance during the intervening years with the *lively dead man*, as I like to call him, the founder of Christian faith. Digging through the layers of doctrinal accretions left by genera-tions of faithful followers, I eventually came face to face with a human being wholly animated by that quality of trust now resonating within. Someone who embodied its potential so thoroughly and uncompromisingly that he made visible the one eliciting such trust. It remains a compelling encounter for, in a way defying explanation, Jesus continues to make his presence felt. Fascination undiminished, inspiration also, he demands my attention and dares me to live out of that trust as authentically and passionately as he did.

Will trust make us better, rescue us from death, draw us into eternity? I cannot say. But trust will relate us aright to those presences beyond us, whose gift is our wholeness and whose promise is our future.

Postscript – An Anatomy of Trust

The past months have yielded many valuable insights into what it means to be human, some of which extend beyond times of illness to characterise our existence more generally. One, in particular, emerges as fundamental. Earlier, I noted how suffering can be a proving experience, stripping away the superficial and inconsequential to expose something of what I referred to as the naked self. Personally, I found this to be a disorientating and distressing process because, in the midst of it, you cannot know what, if anything, will survive. In this respect, suffering is both blinding and revealing. One trait, however, not only endured, but flourished – a capacity for trust. Many, I suspect, will have discovered the same. For this reason, I thought it would be helpful to conclude with a more extended reflection.

The title of this chapter affirms my conviction that trust, far from being tangential, constitutes the architecture of the soul, the inner frame capable of articulating and animating wholesome human being. It does not require much imagination to recognise that, without physical skeletons, our bodies would lack the definition, rigidity and coordination to stand upright, move, communicate, procreate or undertake even the most rudimentary of tasks. In a comparable way, the experience of being a patient has convinced me that without trust we equally struggle to grow into the fullness of our humanity, to inhabit its capacities, constraints and potential creatively, and to help others to do likewise. So let us attend to this anatomy a little more closely.

We begin with the *marrow* running through the whole edifice, the *instinctive quality* of trust. This may appear an incongruous point of departure given many of us find it so demanding, even unnatural. Here it is helpful to draw a distinction between a trusting disposition and the trustworthiness of others. Research into the psychology of child development suggests that whilst the former is innate, the latter is the outcome of experience which can either reinforce or undermine our capacity for trust – trust preserved, builds confidence and relationships; trust betrayed, leaves us diminished, suspicious and tentative; and each has the capacity to impact upon life as a whole, suggesting trust is as intrinsic to our humanity as drawing breath. Starved of air, we suffocate and die; starved of trustworthy presences, we introvert and implode. And whilst a paucity of the former may be more immediately obvious, we wilt in the absence of either.

To appreciate why this is the case, we would do well to attend to trust's *ecstatic feet*. *Ecstasis* is a Greek word meaning 'to be taken beyond ourselves' – hence, ecstasy, the drug and the altered state of consciousness. Trust is no hallucinogen, but it does draw us out of ourselves, into ourselves, by facilitating the formation of enriching relationships through which a fuller sense of self emerges. There is, then, a kind of centrifugal momentum to trust which reflects our desire for growth and expansiveness. For instance, no sooner have we gained even a measure of control over our feet as infants than we're off. In truth, the activity defines our identity as we morph into 'toddlers' – exploring, experiencing, encountering our surroundings with unbridled enthusiasm and untainted innocence. Gradually, through trial and error, consolidation and disillusionment, the passage of time and the seasoning of the character, we learn to temper trust's ecstasis as we discover who and what is trustworthy, whether and where to tread; but even then we never really escape its naivety.

There is something inherently risky about trust. I remember a Sunday school talk on the subject which included the following well-used visual aid. The leader asked for a volunteer. Trustingly, I put up my hand and was summoned to the front. "Stand here," he said reassuringly, "when I ask you, fall backwards and I will catch you before you strike the floor." That sensation of letting go, of trust's exposure, remains with me to this day. It was an apt illustration and one which prepared me for a more urgent and somewhat less contrived experiment in the back of an ambulance that New Year's Eve.

Hands are capable of many things, but trust's hands are open, upturned and empty. They bear its *vulnerability*. In a sense, this is an expression of risk, but of a very particular kind. Let me explain. We might risk investing in the stock market and, if unfortunate, would lose something that was once ours. At worst, it would leave us destitute, but even then the risk relates to our property rather than to our person. By contrast, when we place our trust in the pilot of the plane in which we are travelling or the surgeon preparing to perform an operation on us or the person to whom we are about to say "I will" in church or licensed premises, we lay ourselves bare. For, to varying degrees, trust requires us to place our lives in their hands and, through doing so, we become vulnerable. They may prove trustworthy; they may betray our trust; there is only one way of finding out.

But there is more to vulnerability than entrusting. Sometimes, it is the life of another that rests in trust's palms. The victims of oppression or disaster, the birth of a child, a colleague who confides in us, the neighbour living alone, falling in love, caring for elderly relatives, there are so many scenarios in which our lives are touched by others and trust beckons us to let them in – to let their presence be felt and impact upon us personally.

This quite naturally connects us to trust's *arms of relating*, for vulnerability engenders encounter which can, in turn, blossom into communion. When we are genuinely open to the 'otherness' of other people, as well as the world around us, we escape from that room of mirrors that imperceptibly forms around us, reflecting our impressions and projections of who or what is 'out there'. Trust is the medium through which this takes place and the consequences can be far-reaching. Relationships of commitment are an obvious case in point where we determine to share our lives to some measure – our time and space, memories and thoughts, fears and aspirations, bodies and affections, values and beliefs, families and friends. There is never sufficient grounds for embarking on such an adventure and to do so leaves all parties vulnerable and exposed, yet the mutual expansiveness and enrichment characterising such trusting communion is perhaps the greatest grace life is able to bestow. What is more, it is one that readily overflows into other relationships as our capacity for trust is restored and expanded.

This can, indeed, be a blessing, but covenant relationships characterised by openness are not without challenge and personal cost, as anyone who has endeavoured to maintain a marriage, friendship or partnership or to belong to a family or community of one sort or another will know. This is where trust's *backbone of faithfulness* proves invaluable – the discipline of sustaining vulnerability through time. Nowhere is this more evident than in the practice of forgiveness occasioned by someone exploiting or abusing our trust. The impact of such betrayal can be devastating. Instinctively, we close up and withdraw to protect ourselves from further incursions, tending our wounds. Forgiveness, by contrast, is that counter-intuitive capacity to maintain trust's covenant. To acknowledge the wrong inflicted upon us and to suffer its consequences whilst remaining open to our betrayer. This is a tall order in any circumstance and sometimes should be discouraged, for instance when the forgiveness of children is sought by their abusers as a means of perpetuating abuse. Yet genuine forgiveness, which is a gift the betrayed alone can bestow, possesses unquantifiable potential for catalysing change as well as for restoring, even deepening, fractured relationships.

Thankfully, trust's faithfulness is not always so demanding. Often it finds expression through those rituals and routines constituting the substance of our relationships which may appear inconsequential when viewed in isolation, yet together communicate our ongoing receptiveness to one another: remembering a birthday or anniversary, words of appreciation, preparing a meal, gestures of affection, to mention some of the most obvious examples. Also, through the offering of attention and, with it, a sensitivity for the unexpected – to be surprised by one who has become a familiar, predictable feature within the landscape of our lives. To be struck by their otherness once more.

Which puts us in touch with trust's *sympathetic limbs*. Legs are remarkably versatile appendages enabling us to traverse vast distances across varied terrain and at diverse speeds. With them we can shuffle, walk or run, skip, hop or jump, crouch, swerve or sway, move forwards, backwards or from side to side. Nowhere is their promise more manifest than on the dance floor where, at the bidding of a talented owner, they perform the most intricate of manoeuvres with precision, rhythm and style. They also enable us to dance with someone else – to synchronise, anticipate, respond, to move as one through the unfolding drama of a tango or a waltz. In truth, there can be few more visible demonstrations of sympathy than professional dancers in full flow.

Trust also possesses a pronounced sympathetic strain for, although we may maintain a trusting disposition, it is realised within the concrete instantiations that occur through the course of our relating. Trust emerges in response to, synchronous with and in anticipation of the outworking of another life in as much as it impacts upon ours and vice versa. Trust is not exercised in the abstract, but within the climate of the specific and the particular. It's the means by which we accompany another person and are able to be present with them and for them. Again, this is something that being a patient has taught me. If someone had asked me last December whether I trusted by wife, family, friends, work colleagues, even members of the medical profession, I would have answered in the affirmative with varying degrees of conviction. Now, however, in the light of the intervening months characterised by demonstrations of trustworthiness in the unfolding of an illness, I am able to endorse that judgement with the authority of experience.

Our examination of trust's anatomy is almost complete. We have discovered that trust is *an innate capacity to transcend self through openness and vulnerability, exposing us to the possibility of encounter whilst enabling us to be drawn into relationship, sustain covenant and maintain sympathy.* Hands, arms, feet, legs, spine, marrow. So far, so good, but not all is accounted for. What of the cranium and rib cage, those cathedrals of our being where mind and heart reside? Is this where the analogy breaks down?

I hope not, although this brings us to trust's most mysterious quality which is perhaps best described as an *abiding*, a kind of personal intuiting. At first, it manifests itself as a risky innocence extended towards one eliciting our trust. This yields a certain expansiveness where our trust meets trust and we grow in self-knowledge through encounter. With time, trust beckons us deeper into being-in-relation as we realise aspects of ourselves hitherto undiscovered. This yields an energising confidence in and appreciation of those in whom we trust. They become a part of us and part of us belongs to them. Not in a restricting, static or possessive way; rather, one animating trust's dynamic: an integrity where the sacred of each, their unfathomable otherness, is acknowledged and respected in a communion of mutual entrusting. It is here that our wholeness resides.

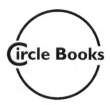

Circle Books

Circle is a symbol of infinity and unity. It's part of a growing list of imprints, including o-books.net and zero-books.net.

Circle Books aims to publish books in Christian spirituality that are fresh, accessible, and stimulating.

Our books are available in all good English language bookstores worldwide. If you can't find the book on the shelves, then ask your bookstore to order it for you, quoting the ISBN and title. Or, you can order online—all major online retail sites carry our titles.

To see our list of titles, please view www.Circle-Books.com, growing by 80 titles per year.

Authors can learn more about our proposal process by going to our website and clicking on Your Company > Submissions.

We define Christian spirituality as the relationship between the self and its sense of the transcendent or sacred, which issues in literary and artistic expression, community, social activism, and practices. A wide range of disciplines within the field of religious studies can be called upon, including history, narrative studies, philosophy, theology, sociology, and psychology. Interfaith in approach, Circle Books fosters creative dialogue with non-Christian traditions.

And tune into MySpiritRadio.com for our book review radio show, hosted by June-Elleni Laine, where you can listen to authors discussing their books.

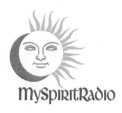

MySpiritRadio